Learn the truth about trans fats

Trans fats, the killer in your food, are found in partially hydrogenated vegetable oil. Partially hydrogenated vegetable oil is completely artificial and bears no chemical, physical, or nutritional resemblance to pure, unadulterated oil.

To food manufacturers, hydrogenated oils are a dream come true because they're inexpensive to manufacture and have an extended "shelf life," allowing for storage without refrigeration.

The National Institute of Health has funded over $100 million on three studies at Harvard University over the past 20 years—the results of which unequivocally prove that the risk of cardiovascular disease correlates to the consumption of trans fats.

TRANS FATS
The Hidden Killer in Our Food

"Judith Shaw uncovers the hidden weapon of mass destruction known as trans fats, a time bomb ticking in every one of us who has succumbed to the lure of processed food. For your sake, and that of your children, you must read this book."
—Oscar London, M.D., author of *Kill as Few Patients as Possible*

Trans Fats

The Hidden Killer In Our Food

Judith Shaw, M.A.

with the assistance of Doris Ober

Foreword by Jeffrey M. Aron, M.D.
University of California, San Francisco

POCKET BOOKS
New York   London   Toronto   Sydney

An *Original* Publication of POCKET BOOKS

POCKET BOOKS, a division of Simon & Schuster, Inc.
1230 Avenue of the Americas, New York, NY 10020

ISBN-13: 978-0-7434-9183-9
ISBN-10:   0-7434-9183-1
First Pocket Books printing May 2004

19 18 17 16 15 14 13 12 11 10

POCKET and colophon are registered trademarks of
Simon & Schuster, Inc.

Cover design by John Vairo Jr.

For information regarding special discounts for bulk purchases,
please contact Simon & Schuster Special Sales at 1-800-456-6798
or business@simonandschuster.com

Manufactured in the United States of America

The ideas, procedures, and suggestions in this book are intended
to supplement, not replace, the medical advice of trained professionals. All matters regarding your health require medical super-
vision. Consult your physician before adopting the medical and/
or dietary suggestions in this book as well as about any condi-
tion that may require diagnosis or medical attention.

The authors and publishers disclaim any liability arising di-
rectly or indirectly from the use of this book.

For Donna Jean Ward
March 1930–March 2003

Contents

Health

PART TWO: ELIMINATING TFAs FROM YOUR HOME AND DIET

Foreword

Judith Shaw has written the dangerous-oil equivalent to Eric Schlosser's *Fast Food Nation* with her book, *Trans Fats: The Hidden Killer in Our Food*. Here is a clear explanation about these dangerous oils, how and why they are produced, and what they do to our health.

She includes practical, everyday methods for shopping and cooking and for eliminating partially hydrogenated oils from our diet. At a time when industry is slowly waking up to the dangers of these oils, this is an invaluable resource to layperson and professional alike.

Our cells are defined by membranes. They not only separate one cell from another; they also determine how cells communicate with each other and govern their internal actions.

Membranes in humans are composed mostly of oils, with some protein and carbohydrate. The oils are continually renewed and replaced. Their composition is affected by the kinds of oils in the diet. Thus the very basic and crucial actions of cells to the proper functioning of the organism depends to a great extent on the oils we consume every day.

Cells must be flexible and be able to change readily in response to signals, such as hormones and triggers of inflammation, or to the pressure of growth from adjacent cells. The oils allow for the proper flexibility or fluidity of the cell membranes and present the proper targets to chemical messengers that coordinate critical body functions.

When partially hydrogenated vegetable oils find their way into our diet, like other oils they are easily incorporated into our cell membranes. Unlike the essential oils in our diet, they stay much longer and change the flexibility of our membranes. The membranes become stiff and lose their ability to signal and respond appropriately to the demands of life. This has the same effect as fine grains of sand dropped into the workings of the most complex Swiss watch: The watch will fail to keep perfect time, then eventually break down completely.

This is what happens to us when we consume partially hydrogenated vegetable oils or trans fats. We develop a state of inflammation that creates a cascade of metabolic horrors with results that can include insulin resistance, obesity, heart disease, autoimmune disease, and depression.

In this book, Judith Shaw has given the reader an invaluable, easily understood insight into everything that should be known about these oils. This work, along with that of other researchers and dedicated physicians and scientists, will do much to change the use of these oils by the food industry, because it will help you, the consumer, make the intelligent choices that will change the demands of the marketplace, the most powerful force that governs industry. As a result, your health will improve, your life will be happier, and the deluge of disease will become less of a threat to us all.

Jeffrey M. Aron, M.D.,
University of California, San Francisco

Author's Note

This is the story of a killer ingredient tucked into most of the food that you, your family, and most other Americans eat. It remains a "secret" ingredient to most Americans, even after ominous warnings from internationally renowned physicians and the Food and Nutrition Board of the Institute of Medicine, our government's adviser on health policy. The hidden ingredient is not something you can see, like a donut, an avocado and tomato sandwich, or a sirloin steak. This killer, originally an unintentional by-product of a manufactured fat, is now slipped into supermarket boxes and packages, fast-food and bakery goodies, to create the mouthfeel of butter and to prolong shelf life. These days there is nothing unintentional about including this manufactured fat in packaged foods. In fact, adding it to our foods has been a deliberate, profit-making decision by the majority of food processors and fast-food giants for at least 20 years. They have gotten you to love the food that kills you. And they know it.

This killer lives inside the manufactured fat you may know by its familiar name, partially hydrogenated vegetable oil. These words appear in small print in the ingredients listing on the millions of wrappers of packaged food produced in the United States, packages you buy at your market and take home to your family. It is also, if one knows to look, listed as an ingredient at fast-food restaurants and neighborhood bakeries. The name of the hidden killer in the partially hydrogenated vegetable oil is trans fatty acid, TFA for short. This book tells how partially hydrogenated vegetable oil, the manufactured fat with TFA, infiltrated the food of our nation and brought about a major transformation in the diet of the world.

This is the story of how it began, how good intentions led the way to an industrial process that creates products responsible for ill-health or death in consumers. It is the story of what happens when capitalism has no rules and science is supported by industry. Odd, is it not, how our government has the power to force the recall of strollers and scooters yet not the power to identify with a cautionary label a poison in our food? Yes, this is the story of the secret you were not supposed to know.

I'm writing this book because of my concern for the impact of manufactured TFAs on our health, our children's health in particular. Heart disease and type 2 diabetes have traditionally been diseases of adulthood; now they are diseases that begin in childhood. Children are the most vulnerable victims of advertising and marketing. Moving into adolescence with their own disposable dollars, children become the principal consumers of foods with hydrogenated vegetable oils, snacking away at the cellophane packages and fast foods that have become a thirty billion dollar American habit. This habit cuts across economic and social class lines. Consuming foods with hydrogenated oils (chips, cookies, crackers, muffins, donuts, candy, fast food—to name just a few) has become a national pastime, a cultural institution. According to the Food and Drug Administration (FDA), fully half of packaged cereals, cold or hot, contain partially hydrogenated vegetable oils. Even school lunches may contain partially hydrogenated vegetable oils, and partially hydrogenated vegetable oils *always* contain the killer ingredient TFA. A tragic piece of this story is that no one knows just how much of this poison each of us or our children eat; hydrogenated vegetable oils are the food industry's Trojan horse. The FDA has mandated that trans fatty acids be listed in the "nutrition facts" section of package labels (along with other fats that are already listed), but that regulation does not go into full effect until January of 2006.

The good news is that you don't have to wait until 2006 to eliminate trans fats from your diet. You can stop feeding your family TFAs now. This book will tell you everything you need to know about partially hydrogenated vegetable oils and manufactured TFAs and their dangers. You'll learn now where the killer ingredient hides. You'll become an expert on what's tainted and what's not, in the marketplace and in restaurants.

The first part of the book shares the kind of background material that I learned while investigating this subject: a little science, a little history, the political story, the health implications.

Part two will help you recognize what foods contain manufactured TFAs and show you how to choose well when you shop. Ideas for converting to a TFA-free household will help your family make the transition to a healthier lifestyle without sacrificing much more than brand loyalty. Appendixes contain a comprehensive list of TFA-free brands and foods, a resource list of books and websites, and medical references.

As you read along, you will learn what many dedicated scientists and medical researchers have discovered in their laboratories and learned from their carefully investigated studies. They have gracious and generously shared their knowledge with me, in person, on the telephone, or through their writings. I wrote this book so that you in turn may benefit from the wisdom and dedication of the men and women who have worked long and toilsome hours to bring forth this truth, a truth generally hidden, discredited, or resisted. Until now.

Judith Shaw
January, 2004

In which we drive down a main street in America . . .

Drive east on Wilshire Boulevard, make a left onto Fairfax. If it's winter, you'll see the trees and lush green of the Hollywood hills. Pressed against that backdrop and a little off to the left is the glass front of the superstore 99 Cents Only, stacked with merchandise—an organized jumble of sodas, giant packages of candy bars, crackers, cookies, cakes, daily specials, and not so daily specials all beckoning the shopper to stop, shop, and carry home some of the hundreds of familiar food brands that are offered at hugely discounted prices.

Here customers fill their carts with pudding, soups, chips, dips, and donuts then browse the aisles for soda, corn-syrup-sweetened fruit drinks and extras like party favors, Halloween masks, nail polish, panties and brassieres, and men's undershirts. The store's daily specials usually include a dinner food bargain, like the one I see today: Morton's Vegetable Pie with Chicken.

99 Cents Only stores and others of its kind offer shoppers a mostly good deal, from an economic point of view. The

bad part of the deal is that much of the food—including the Morton's Vegetable Pie with Chicken special—is loaded with partially hydrogenated vegetable oils, a manufactured fat that harbors an ingredient that kills: the ingredient known as trans fatty acid.

PART ONE

Background

On July 10, 2002, the government's adviser on health policy, the Institute of Medicine at the National Academy of Sciences, reported that Americans are eating foods contaminated with dangerous levels of manufactured trans fatty acids, an ingredient that has *no safe level for human consumption:* in the words of the report, an "upper intake level of zero." About 40 percent of supermarket foods contain trans fat. The FDA says that it's in 95 percent of cookies, 80 percent of frozen breakfast foods, 75 percent of snacks and chips, 70 percent of cake mixes, and almost half of all cereals. The packaged products it lists with the most trans fat include vegetable shortening, donuts, stick margarine, french fries, and microwave popcorn.

The principal outcome of the Institute of Medicine's announcement in 2002 is that the FDA formally instituted a labeling requirement mandating that by 2006 all manufactured packaged foods will indicate the presence of this killer ingredient. It has been nine years since the FDA was first petitioned (1994) to do this, and it has been more than four years since the FDA first announced its plan (November 12, 1999) to have trans fatty acids included on nutrition labels. Yes, it has been slow work.

The irony and tragedy is that a lone chemist in Baltimore and several concerned medical researchers have been documenting the potential dangers of this killer fatty acid in our food for the past twenty years. Moreover, since the early 1990s, scientists and physicians at Harvard University and other influential institutions worldwide have published evidence that absolutely implicates manufactured trans fatty acids in our continuing epidemics of heart disease, type 2 diabetes, and obesity. What they discovered and wrote about and what consumer advocates and researchers pleaded with the FDA to do years ago should have alarmed all practicing physicians and everyone else—if only anyone had paid attention . . .

Science

Chapter One

The Hydrogenated Bomb

Partially hydrogenated vegetable oil is a manufactured substitute for true fats, such as butter or unprocessed vegetable oil. In this manufactured fat lives the killer, trans fatty acid.

Partially hydrogenated vegetable oil is the fat in much of the packaged food you purchase—the United States Department of Agriculture (USDA) says it's in 40 percent of the food on grocery store shelves—and in much of the fast food, bakery goods, and take-out food you eat. It's a fat with calories, the same number as other fats, and the mouthfeel of butter.

There the similarity ends. Partially hydrogenated vegetable oil contains the killer you have been reading about in your newspapers, manufactured trans fatty acid (TFA). The TFA in partially hydrogenated vegetable oil is the stuff that the Institute of Medicine, on July 10, 2002, declared a serious danger to the [cardiac] health of our nation with a "tolerable upper intake level of zero."

Partially hydrogenated vegetable oil was first used in the early 1900s as a substitute for the beef fat (oleo) and skim milk of the original margarine recipe. Hydrogenating vegetable oil produced a less expensive, cleaner looking, cleaner smelling, longer lasting alternative and a perfect cooking substitute. But it is completely artificial and bears no chemical or physical resemblance to the pure, unadulterated vegetable oil that is its raw material. For the last ninety years, partially hydrogenated vegetable oil has graduated from being the artificial fat source for margarine to being the major food-manufacturing fat in the United States.

Partially hydrogenated vegetable oils, which do not exist in nature and never have, always contain the manufactured killer fatty acid, TFA.

How Hydrogenated Oil Is Manufactured

To manufacture partially hydrogenated vegetable oil, the first step is to crush soybeans, corn, sunflower seeds, rapeseed (commonly known as canola), safflower seeds, or cottonseed, which yields fresh, pure vegetable oils that have their own particular valuable properties—but not for long. The oils readied for hydrogenation are then refined with chemical solvents: deodorizing agents and bleaches. This initial process begins the destruction of the original oil's good-for-you fatty acids.

As the process of hydrogenation begins, a small amount of a metal catalyst is added to the oil. This is usually nickel, a substance that quickens the chemical reaction. The hydrogenation process is completed by adding hydrogen gas under very high pressure and very high heat. This "cooking" changes the molecular configuration of the once benign vegetable oil, creating a substance that is plastic and thicker and can hold a shape, no longer an oil at all. The manufactured product is solid at room temperature. About to be part of a manufactured cookie, cake, or chicken nugget, it looks like fat—semisoft butter or hardened chicken fat. You know this reconfigured, manufactured fat as two common market products, margarine and vegetable shortening (most commonly Crisco). In packaged foods it's listed under "Ingredients" as partially hydrogenated vegetable oil. In some instances, partially hydrogenated vegetable oil is camouflaged as shortening or margarine.

Unfortunately, when many consumers who do read ingredient labels on packages see the words vegetable oil, even when it is part of the phrase partially hydrogenated, their minds read "healthy." Even the managers of some individual outlets of fast-food businesses, such as Krispy Kreme and McDonald's, have been educated by senior management to believe that the hydrogenated vegetable oils used in their products are healthy replacements for unprocessed vegetable oils, butter, or lard. Moreover, many health-conscious consumers, some of the hundred million who went online in 2001 to seek health-related information, according to the *Journal of the American Medical Association*, are frequently unaware that their wheat bread, their granola bars, their "special" sauces, their bran muffins, even many of the restaurant foods they eat have significant amounts of partially hydrogenated vegetable oils. In fact, partially hydrogenated vegetable oil is just a friendly sounding euphemism for the killer molecule, TFA.

Why Food Manufacturers Love Hydrogenated Oils

To food manufacturers, hydrogenated oils are a dream come true. They are inexpensive to manufacture, they're flavorless—scent and taste are added later—and they have a long shelf life. Shelf life is the length of time a box of crackers, cookies, chips, cereal, bread, or pizza crust can sit on a grocer's shelf before becoming stale. Foods made with partially hydrogenated vegetable oils have an indeterminate storage time or shelf life. Sometimes it's years.

In a fast-food restaurant, it is the hydrogenation of the frying oil that gives your fries, fish sticks, and chicken nuggets that nice crisp crunch. It's hydrogenation that allows the cooking oil for frying to be reused repeatedly and makes it unnecessary to refrigerate many salad dressings and sauces.

Yes, hydrogenation is a dream for the food industry and agribusiness, but it's a nightmare for your health and that of your family.

Chapter Two

The Killer
Molecule, TFA

The recipe for hydrogenation—deodorized and bleached vegetable oil, high heat, hydrogen, a metal catalyst—brought about a miracle product. It also created the killer, trans fatty acid.

All partially hydrogenated vegetable oils contain the by-product TFA. If you read the words, "partially hydrogenated vegetable oil" on packaged food or an ingredient list, there never needs to be a question in your mind about whether TFAs are in that food. They are.

It is important to note that a special kind of TFA does exist in nature and has always been part of the food supply. This TFA comes from ruminant animals (cattle, sheep, goats, deer), characteristically animals with a four-compartment stomach and that chew their cud of regurgitated, partially digested food. Natural TFAs, therefore, show up, in very small amounts, in dairy products and meat. But these natural TFAs have different chemical configurations (different isomers) from the manufactured version. Chemically reconfigured, artificial TFAs fool your cells. They are pretenders, hardening cell walls and impeding flexibility and mobility.

Manufactured TFA molecules wreak havoc with our cells.

They take up cell space, establishing a surplus of the wrong kind of fatty acid in our bodies. As TFAs play politics with the basic underpinnings of our bodies, the integrity of our cell membranes are wrecked. Over time, as cells continue to be invaded with TFAs, they become less effective, compromised in their capacity to sustain optimum health.

That TFA poisoning is cumulative over time makes its effects hard to see and harder to comprehend. There is no immediate visible disaster, no fever, rash, vomiting, no pain; the process is like smoking tobacco, with its carcinogenic tars, or drinking water with pesticide residue: The resulting disease takes years to show up.

Health and nutrition information changes so often that you may be thinking that TFAs sound like just one more in a long string of things that aren't good for us. That, like so many other foods, they will one day be proven to be good for us or at least not as dangerous as what you've read so far.

No such possibility. That will never be. There is no gray area here, no upside to this artificial, plasticlike substance, no bodily function that it enhances. Manufactured TFAs can be nothing but detrimental to your body. And they compromise our bodies at the most basic level—cellular function. From that point on, our health is in jeopardy.

The good news: TFAs will be eliminated from your cells when you no longer eat foods that contain them. Given the chance, healthy fatty acids will eventually replace them, and normal cellular function will be restored. Unfortunately, structural damage already done can't be undone, but it can be halted—and that process starts the moment you stop consuming TFAs.

What Foods Contain TFAs?

Processed and packaged foods contain manufactured TFAs to give the foods longer shelf life. Look into your cupboards or refrigerator or freezer. Any package that lists partially hydrogenated vegetable oil in its ingredients contains TFAs. Many hamburger buns, frozen fries, pot pies, frozen pizzas, tacos, cereals, and pie crusts contain TFAs. The baby and toddler food sold in boxes and jars may have them. Arrowroot Cookies from Gerber and Nabisco's Zwieback Toast and Animal Crackers have them. Licorice, cheesecake, cornbread mixes, and brownies may have them. Even cholesterol free and low-fat crackers frequently have them.

TFAs are found in many muffins, donuts, cookies, rolls, and pies. They're in a substantial number of the pastries at all 4,126 Starbucks across the nation. TFAs exist not only at fast-food stops but in any restaurant kitchen where preserving the longevity of cooking oils and partially prepared fried and grilled foods is the primary consideration.

TFAs are often hiding in your salad dressings and your candy bars. They may be in your favorite fried potato skins. TFAs may be in stove-top mixes, frankfurter rolls, packaged bread crumbs, and stuffings. TFAs may be doubly camouflaged on some packages as "shortening," as "vegetable shortening," or "hardened vegetable oil." Any baked good or packaged food with margarine in it or one that suggests the use of stick margarine to prepare it is, or becomes, full of TFAs. TFAs may be in the croutons in your Caesar salad, in your fried crab sushi, your egg and muffin. TFAs may be in your blueberry scone or in the bread of your tuna salad sandwich. TFAs may be in the sauce on barbequed chicken or ribs. Most probably, your eggs and hash browns at your favorite lunch counter are cooked in them. Even the new good-for-your-heart spread, Benecol, has them.

Where Else?

Most stick margarines are full of TFAs, and some of the tubs have them as well. Snacks like Quaker Cereal Bars, Pepperidge Farm Goldfish,* Lunchables, and Oreos have them. Granola bars, crackers, cookies, chips, dips, cheese crackers, and flat breads may have them. They may be in canned or freshly made soups, frozen sauced vegetables, and pancake and waffle mixes. Manufactured TFAs lurk in take-out salads, apple pies, and stir-fries. They may be in canned french fried onions and in the fried onions at fast-food stops. They are in the sugar-free candy made expressly for diabetics. Bread sticks and Halloween treats may have them. They are most certainly in nondairy coffee creamer and frequently in egg substitutes. Peanut butters and packaged nut treats may have them. Hospital patients are served them. Airplane food is infested with them.

Hydrogenated vegetable oil is the fat of choice for many restaurant deep fryers, sauté pans, and grills. Even some name brand ice creams, like Ben & Jerry's, have them. Orville Redenbacher "quality" popcorn uses them, so do most other microwave popcorns.

No cooking, baking, or frying, domestic or commercial, *requires* the use of partially hydrogenated vegetable oil. TFAs, the fatty acids that no human can metabolize and manufactured in vast quantities around the world, exist solely for commercial profit.

---

* On February 17, 2004, *The New York Times* reported that the Campbell's soup company, the parent company of Pepperidge Farm, announced that it was planning to eliminate TFAs from its Goldfish recipe. As this book goes to press, however, Pepperidge Farm Goldfish still contain TFAs.

History

Chapter Three

Hydrogenation: An Idea Whose Time Had Come

Originally, partially hydrogenated vegetable oil was a gift to every household, an innocent and brilliant entrepreneurial invention. At the time there was no evidence that the changes brought about by the chemical cleaning and hydrogenation of vegetable oils were harmful.

Hydrogenation was a French idea. How incongruous that a country known for baby radishes, just-born greens, infant lamb, perfectly ripe cheese, sublime soufflés would spawn an artificial fat, a gastrological tragedy upon the world.

What was happening in France at the time that led to hydrogenation? What made hydrogenation an idea whose time had come?

The Historical Perspective

By the middle of the nineteenth century, the Industrial Revolution had created a massive migration to manufacturing centers throughout Europe. While factories boomed across the continent, the population suffered from what a migration surge usually creates—high prices, food shortages, housing scarcity, poor sanitation and health.

The mid-nineteenth century was the time of the Second Empire in France. Napoleon III's politics reaped vast material and social benefits for the country—in some places.

The rise of urban wealth and the migration of a rural population seeking its fortune through industrialization combined to cause severe nutritional deprivation in cities. While the new middle class could afford extravagant prices, a new class of people found themselves impoverished.

One food the working classes could barely afford was animal fat—beef, butter, poultry fat, and lard, from pigs. The scarcity of lard meant the loss of an essential cooking and baking ingredient.

While the upper classes and individuals in highly skilled occupations thrived in central Paris and in other major industrial centers, artisans and the assembly-line workers were frequently in distress. One slum outside the capital city was called the Siberia of Paris for the severity of its conditions. Living places—ghettos reserved for workers in Paris and in manufacturing centers all over Europe—were often squalid neighborhoods of disenchantment and disillusionment, where men and women worked twelve-hour days at crippling labor on an inadequate diet. In Paris in the 1870s, many people lived in poverty that verged on starvation.

Hunger and poverty were not an exclusively French phenomenon. In England, it was a sign of prosperity if a working man's family was able to serve bread at a meal. For a hundred years, the staple food for the Dutch working family was the potato. The common French blue-collar diet at the time was soup; a miner's family might eat beef five times a year; a factory worker might eat pork scraps but only rarely. Butter existed only in dreams. In the last half of the nineteenth century in the United States, New York City was a crowded slum rampant with disease, teeming with the poor, the uneducated, the hungry, poised for terrifying municipal riots and gang warfare.

European governments, especially France, urged scientists to look for solutions to its food problems. If they could curtail spoilage, it would go a long way toward eliminating the shortages that led to despair, illness, and crime. Food substitutes and food preservation were priorities.

Napoleon III offered outright financial gifts to French scientists, which encouraged and enabled a climate of scientific investigation. And so it was in France in 1869 that a chemist named Hippolyte Mège-Mouriès invented a product composed completely of animal products—beef tallow and milk—that eventually revolutionized the eating habits of the world. It was the miracle he called margarine.

The Invention of Margarine

Mège-Mouriès used an acid called margaric to make margarine. This was a fatty acid that had been isolated by another French chemist, Michel-Eugène Chevreul, in 1813. Chevreul named his pearly, lustrous acid after the Greek word for pearl, *margaron.* "Oleo," from the Latin *oleum* (oil), was attached as a prefix to the word margarine and was commonly part of the name until after World War II.

The first margarine did not resemble the butter or lard it was intended to replace. It was an unattractive brownish color, was prone to becoming rancid, and had the unfortunate fragrance of rendered meat parts. Not until 1910 was margarine made of nonmeat products.

While the new margarine did not solve the shortage of

beef and pork fats and of butter in Europe, what made it popular was that it was more affordable. Most important, it behaved somewhat like butter or lard in cooking.

Even though affordable, the original margarine was expensive to produce. A new focus became crucial: how to replace expensive, hard-to-render animal products with something that was cheaper to manufacture and would not spoil. Scientists looked for a better alternative.

Could vegetable oils substitute for animal fats? Of course it was thought of and was an attractive idea, but it needed the invention of hydrogenation to produce that cleaner, sweeter, rancidity-resistant margarine that has become ubiquitous in America and the world. And that time hadn't quite come yet.

Genius at Work

In the meantime, the French government continued allocating large grants to its relatively unknown chemists to encourage food-related inventions. It was during this time, for instance, that Louis Pasteur discovered that infectious disease is caused by germs, that organisms live in air but do not originate in air.

In devising the basic rules of sterilization, Pasteur also revolutionized surgery and obstetrics through his understanding that the two-thousand year-old notion of spontaneous generation (that life arises spontaneously from organic materials) was erroneous. This discovery led to the identification of germs, which in turn led to a firm and powerful advocacy for hand washing in the surgical theatre and for women's confinement. While hand washing at childbirth had been strongly advocated by Ignaz Semmelweis in Vienna and his physician colleague Oliver Wendell Holmes in Boston as early as the 1840s, there was only the proof of their own research, which consisted of counting the dead, washing hands, and then counting the survivors. Mainstream scientists and physicians needed the evidence Pasteur showed them.

Pasteur also revealed the world of viruses through his work with rabies. Among other phenomenal contributions to medicine and microbiology, he demonstrated that the diseases of wine could be controlled by heating the wine to 55 degrees Celsius. This process became known as pasteurization and continues to safeguard many industry-packaged beverages today, the most famous, of course, being milk.

Not much later, in 1899, the Frenchman Auguste Gaulin patented a homogenizer pump to mechanically disperse or homogenize the fat globules of pasteurized milk. Before the century ended, the next food-manufacturing miracle— hydrogenation of oils—was theorized by two French chemists, Paul Sabatier and Jean-Baptiste Senderens.

They discovered that there was more hydrogen in solid animal fats than in vegetable oils. What would happen, they wondered, if they added hydrogen to vegetable oil? Might its addition harden vegetable oil so it could be used in the manufacture of margarine? Could this result in a cheaper product?

It was a German scientist, Willhelm Normann, who tried the theory first and invented hydrogenation. He patented the process in 1902, and an industry was born. The first (and least expensive) vegetable oil to be hydrogenated for margarine in the United States was cottonseed. It lost popularity because of the pesticides used to kill the boll weevil. By 1925, coconut oil had become the principal fat. After World War II, corn oil dominated in the United States until soybeans became the major source of hydrogenated oils worldwide. By the 1950s, hydrogenated oils in the form of margarine had become entrenched as America's most popular spread.

Crisco: a Brief History

In 1913, Procter & Gamble, the makers of Ivory Soap, began to market Crisco. It was the first edible food product, other than margarine, manufactured with hydrogenated oils. Along with margarine, the all-pure, all-white hydrogenated Crisco fat eventually changed the cooking habits of every North American household and every North American restaurant and the diets of the world.

Crisco was introduced as an alternative to animal fats, an innovative cooking fat more economical than butter, "a scientific discovery which [would] affect every kitchen in America," according to the Procter & Gamble company magazine, "Moonbeams." As the story goes, William Cooper Procter walked into the office of a man who had been in the cooking oil business most of his life and tossed a hard white block onto his desk. "There is some cottonseed oil," Mr. Procter said.

"Right then and there," the magazine story continues, "today's entire hydrogenated vegetable oil industry was born."

The first Crisco came onto the marketplace in round, handmade, wooden crates, lovely enough to qualify as collector's items today. No expense seemed to be too extravagant in the marketing process. Teams of home economists descended on the largest auditoriums across the country to offer Crisco cooking demonstrations. Distinctive blue-and-white cans eventually became its trademark and its miracle product flew off grocery store shelves into pantries across the country.

Because Crisco was pure vegetable oil and contained no animal products, it could be market-projected not just to traditional American homes but also to Jewish households, Islamic households, vegetarian households—any home with dietary restrictions on meat or combining of meat and dairy products. The prospects were enormous. Among Procter & Gamble's promotional efforts were Crisco cookbooks for the general public and ones specifically written for Japanese, Jewish, or Philippine households. There were, among many titles, *A Cookery Course in 13 Chapters; 24 Pies Men Like; Candies and Confections; Crisco Recipes for the Jewish Housewife; Recipes for Everyday;* and of course *School Lunches.*

Crisco surged in popularity as a result of animal fat rationing during World War I. By the end of the war in 1918, Crisco was a well-known household staple. Its second surge came during World War II, again as a result of butter and meat rationing. By the time the war ended in 1945, it was, along with another product called Spry, the universal home-kitchen cooking and baking fat in American homes and was an essential ingredient in school lunches, hospital food, and railroad dining car grills.

By the 1950s, at about the same time the American Heart Association announced that the United States was in the midst of an epidemic of coronary heart disease with an as yet unknown cause, Crisco was everywhere in America. You could cook, fry, and bake with Crisco. Its whiteness was touted as purity. After it was opened, it could be kept in the can it came in and didn't need to be refrigerated. It was odorless. A major advertising message was that Crisco was 100% pure vegetable fat, not a product that was part water, like butter. Crisco appealed to everyone.

Even though the trend and preoccupation in urban and sophisticated suburban America is toward recipe acquisition and nutritional excellence—and less fat—take a look at the shelves where you shop today. Crisco and margarine are still some of the most easily recognized products in the market. Today, Crisco alone has $350 million in annual sales.

In fact, since the 1970s, most of the food purchased in the market, picked up at takeouts, selected in bakeries, or eaten in fast-food places has contained one type or another of manufactured partially hydrogenated vegetable oils: margarine, Crisco, or just plain hydrogenated cooking oils.

In 2001, Procter & Gamble sold Crisco to the J. M. Smucker Company ("With a name like Smucker's, it has to be good!"), thus ending its ninety-year affiliation with vegetable shortening. But not the nation's. At least not yet.

Chapter Four

Two Events That Supported the Growth of an Industry

By 1956, Crisco, the ubiquitous vegetable shortening for home cooking and baking, and margarine, the spread of choice for millions of Americans, were the major sources of manufactured trans fatty acids in food.

Between the beginning of 1956 and the end of 1958, two events had a profound effect on the hydrogenation industry and contributed to its becoming, by 2001, the fourth-largest food-manufacturing process in the world.

Event Number 1: The Interstate Highway System

In 1956, Congress passed legislation to build the interstate highway system, which by linking the forty-eight contiguous states with state-of-the-art roadways forever changed how Americans would shop, commute, and eat. The interstate did for the country what the freeways had already done for Southern California.

In his 2001 book, *Fast Food Nation*, Eric Schlosser talks

about southern California's car culture, already in place in the forties. The roadways linking small towns around burgeoning San Bernadino, Anaheim, and Los Angeles had already welcomed, Schlosser says, the world's first motel and first drive-in bank. By 1948, the brothers Richard and Maurice McDonald had opened the first fast-food assembly-line service system that revolutionized the eating habits and the food itself of American families.

The interstate highway system took forty years to complete, each year connecting more and more small towns and obscure counties to each other and to the rest of the nation. It was a time of major transformation in American life. One can't but suppose that the inspiration for the interstate, for the future of automobile travel, was the extravagant and futuristic superhighway modeled for the public at the New York World's Fair of 1939–40. Men and women who were young adults or children then can remember the excitement of seeing the prototypes. The dream was of roads that would lead anywhere, concrete roads called highways (roads above the land) for automobiles to carry Americans with ease and splendor to work and play. Since then, over four million miles of public roadway crisscrossing America have given birth to accessible beaches and parks, suburban communities, central marketplaces, agonizing commutes, a massive trucking industry, and the fast-food stops and convenience stores that feed Americans during their vacations, lunch hours, and time-outs. Two hundred million cars, trucks, and motorcycles populate these roads, said Tom Lewis, author of *Divided Highways: Building the Interstate Highways, Transforming American Life.*

With exit ramps as destinations, with the commute as a way of life, with the brilliant innovation of turning fast-food drive-ins into gathering and dining places and malls into strolling and noshing avenues, the new industry of the hydrogenation of vegetable oil found another niche. In addition to making life easier for consumers with drive-ins and take-out food stops, the interstate highway system enabled the food industry to easily transport merchandise across and around the country.

Manufactured hydrogenated oils, which gave long life to margarine and vegetable shortenings like Crisco, could be used to preserve the processed packaged foods being trucked across the country to supermarkets and eating places. Unlike butter, the manufactured hydrogenated vegetable fat in crackers and cookies, precooked french fries and pot pies, buns, muffins, salad dressings, chicken legs, and fish filets ensured that a product that started out in New Jersey would still be fresh when it got to Washington state and for months and years to come. It would preserve foods shipped across the seas.

And there was another benefit to partially hydrogenated vegetable oils' partnership with the interstate highway. The highway made it possible to carry brand names across the country and eventually around the world. It familiarized whole populations with nationally advertised food products that they could count on to look and taste the same wherever they were purchased. Today the brand names you find in a mall in Boston are not dissimilar from those you find in Berlin. Today we can travel from New York to Miami, from Austin to Minneapolis, and count on the familiar logo of McDonald's and Burger King, Taco Bell and Chili's, Safeway or Albertsons.

Nowhere need we be out of touch with what has become commonplace in our neighborhood. If a traveler is hungry, there is a place to eat in San Francisco with the same accustomed menu as a place in St. Louis or Charleston, Toronto or London. Today, as Eric Schlosser notes, Americans can stop to eat at their choice of two hundred thousand familiar fast-food places along the highway. Others stop at market centers and delicatessens to choose among thousands and thousands of packages and takeouts for the evening meal.

Life is easier with these selections to choose from. But the fat in most burger buns and chips and in many of the prepared take-out foods we know is partially hydrogenated vegetable oil, within which lies trans fatty acid.

Event Number 2:
The Food Additives Amendment

The second event that effectively strengthened the development of the hydrogenation industry occurred on September 6, 1958, when the (FDA) enacted the Food Additives Amendment. It was intended to protect Americans from potentially dangerous substances used in the manufacture of food. It states: "A food shall be deemed to be adulterated if it bears or contains any poisonous or deleterious substance which may render it injurious to health."

But as I discovered in a telephone conversation in February 2002 with George Pauli, director of the Office of Food Additive Safety, food additives in use before 1958—as with partially hydrogenated vegetable oils—did not require FDA approval. Even though the code continues to state that "Foods . . . must be reexamined in the light of current scientific information . . . if their use is to be continued," the food additive safety office has ignored the last twelve years of medical documentation, inquiry and public concern about trans fats. In the same telephone conversation, Dr. Pauli told me that he was unaware of any danger from the trans fatty acids in partially hydrogenated vegetable oil. In fact, he said, he had not heard of them.

I'll bet he has now. What matters is that under the umbrella provided by the FDA, the industry that feeds us the killer trans fatty acids still flourishes. Americans spend 90 percent of their food money on processed foods. And yet, eating packaged food and fast foods in the United States has become high-risk behavior. What happened? Who stopped looking out for us?

Oil Politics

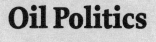

Chapter Five

Why It Took So Long to Learn the Truth About TFAs

Back in the late 1970s, a biochemist named Mary Enig and a few concerned physicians began to question whether there were adverse effects from manufactured trans fatty acids on the human body. Unfortunately, it was years before the people who should have listened did.

By the 1950s heart disease was the leading cause of mortality in the United States, with half a million deaths a year. Before most of us knew to question what a big alteration—like adding hydrogenated vegetable oil to our diet—would do to our hearts or other major bodily systems, a diet that substituted margarine and Crisco for butter and other saturated (animal) fats had become de rigueur. Most Americans had never thought about nutritional health. (Nutrition wasn't even integrated into the course work in medical schools until the 1990s.) It took several decades—until 2002, in fact—before our Institute of Medicine publicly revealed the TFA assault on human hearts.

Why? Because corporate agribusiness exerted pressure on government officials. The powerful edible oil lobby and politicians from farming states drew shut a curtain of secrecy to conceal the startling news that manufactured trans fatty acids raised the levels of the heart-damaging LDL cholesterol and lowered those of the beneficial HDL cholesterol.

The Blame Game: Butter, Red Meat, and Eggs

So what was causing the surge in the rate of heart disease in America? Throughout the 1950s and 1960s, Americans were told the culprit was saturated fat—animal fat—the kind of fat that is dominant in butter, red meat, and eggs. (Learn more about saturated and unsaturated fats in chapter 11.) We were told by the experts then that the epidemic proportions of coronary disease could be halted if the country united against butter, red meat, and eggs. However, funding the research that seemed to unequivocally "prove" the connection between heart disease and diets high in saturated fats were companies such as Procter & Gamble (makers of Crisco), Mazola and Wesson (corn oil), and Fleishmann's (margarine)—the very food giants who stood to benefit most from their conclusions. Today that proof, the structure of the experimentations in those papers that declared saturated fat the culprit and the cognitive leaps made by the researchers, are widely questioned and criticized by scientists and medical researchers.

In his illuminating and well-researched article for *Science* magazine in March 2001, "The Soft Science of Dietary Fat," the science writer Gary Taubes elaborates on the role government had, and still has, in the endorsement of the maintenance of the saturated-fat theory of heart disease; how it was blindly accepted by physicians and the public as the truth, even though it was absolutely lacking in scientific rigor. Taubes illustrates how government policy can affect our health and our behavior with an educational campaign that eventually becomes, as Lillian Cheung, director of health promotion and communication at Harvard has pointed out, "an advertising campaign for [an] industry."

Ironically, at the precise time in the 1950s that saturated fat (butter, meat, eggs) was designated the villain in heart disease, USDA figures showed that butter consumption in the United States had actually dropped to *one-quarter* of what it had been at the turn of the century while consumption of hydrogenated vegetable oil margarine had risen 200 percent, *four times* what it had been in 1900. We were already eating less butter and much more margarine. And yet this information, which seems to clearly contradict the popular idea that escalating rates of heart disease were a result of increases in saturated fats, received scant notice. Matthew Gillman, M.D., a professor of medicine at Harvard University, in a 1997 paper in *Epidemiology* reported, ". . . a rise in coronary heart disease incidence with increasing margarine consumption but little association with butter intake . . . trans fatty acids of vegetable origin conferred a higher risk than those of [butter]."

Not that there weren't scientists straining to be heard. Mary Enig, Ph.D., a Baltimore chemist, began her investigations into TFAs in the late 1970s at the University of Baltimore. Her work, for which she received no federal or food industry support, showed that the addition of hydrogenated vegetable oil caused interrupted life patterns and lowered disease resistance. Initially ridiculed, today she is considered one of the seminal thinkers in the field of trans fats. Fortunately, over time she was joined by a large cohort of renowned scientists, physicians, and investigators who by the early 1990s were publishing their findings on the correlation of TFAs in our diet to heart disease and other health conditions of our time.

But back to the 1950s . . . Several national educational campaigns in the 1950s and 1960s endorsed both margarine and corn oil for the kitchen, supporting the saturated-fat theory of heart disease. These campaigns were not only promoted by the industries that would benefit financially (like the margarine and vegetable oil industries), they were also supported by the federal government and its newly founded American Heart Association. By the 1960s these campaigns were hugely successful. Instead of butter, margarine had become the spread of choice from Park Avenue dining room tables to suburban kitchens, from winter vacation hotels to summer camp sites, on Hollywood movie sets and Beverly Hills patios, in restaurants and diners in every city and town in the country. In many places, it still is.

Urban and suburban, the new diet of the 1950s that was to stave off heart disease swept the nation. Instead of baking with butter, Americans became addicts of the vegetable shortenings, Crisco and Spry. We ate white meat chicken instead of red meat and had breakfasts of synthetic eggs manufactured with hydrogenated vegetable oils. Real eggs, which had once been known as a perfect food, became a memory for saturated-fat-causes-heart-disease advocates. Without realizing it, Americans had become the subjects of a vast national experiment.

Massive amounts of money from government sources and food consortiums supported the new science, and there was no embarrassment on the part of professional recipients for taking honoraria and becoming spokesmen for industry. According to Mary Enig, medical journals, such as *JAMA*, the journal of the American Medical Association, ran ads for Wesson corn oil as a cholesterol depressant during this period. William Castelli, a physician who directed the world-famous Framingham Heart Study, endorsed Puritan corn oil; so did Dr. Antonio Gotto Jr. when he was president of the American Heart Association. Dr. Gotto's personal endorsement was mailed to physicians on the letterhead of the DeBakey Heart Center of the Baylor College of Medicine.

The influence of these physicians was profound. Their promotional advocacy and the endorsements by science and government prompted other doctors to encourage their patients to drastically modify their eating habits. Margarine was the new prescription. There seemed to be no dissenting voice, and the American public had no reason to be skeptical.

Preparing Americans to take on the scourge of heart disease was complete; the country was mobilized. Then President Dwight D. Eisenhower had a heart attack, thrusting heart disease out of the hush-hush of the living room and into the public domain. Radio, television, and print media examined the status of the disease in excruciating detail. The epidemic proportions of heart attack were frightening; everyone now knew someone who had had one.

The heart disease epidemic was reminiscent to many Americans of the treacherous poliomyelitis epidemic of the 1930s and 1940s that afflicted so many. Until the polio vaccine was invented, polio had for years caused families to shun swimming pools and crowded beaches; fearful parents bundled their children off to safe summer camps, away from the cities, and themselves migrated to the desert for untainted air. The memory of the polio menace probably made it easier to mobilize against the heart disease epidemic, to get behind a campaign to once again save our lives. We needed a heart disease hero; it looked as if it were vegetable oil and hydrogenated fat.

As we changed our diets, food manufacturers and a nation of housewives and doctors embraced the supposed heart-safe fats instead of butter, grilling our food in it and baking it into uncountable numbers of goodies. No one at the time, not even the corn, safflower, and up-and-coming soybean processors, could imagine how big the eventual hydrogenated marketplace would become.

By the end of the 1950s, with the new saturated-fat guidelines in place (which amounted to "don't eat them"), numbers for healthy cholesterol levels a matter of public interest, and the American Heart Association's launch of a prudent diet (white meat chicken, synthetic eggs, and corn oil for cooking, and margarine for spreading) for all, we should have been in shape to resist cardiac disease. But our epidemic of heart disease did *not* abate during the fifty years of saturated-fat gospel. Instead, Americans who did not yet have heart disease were becoming an endangered species.

Even now—even after the publication of a large body of research and with the Institute of Medicine's announcing a "a positive linear trend between [TFA] intake and LDL cholesterol [the damaging one] and increased risk of [coronary heart disease] with a tolerable upper intake level of [food manufactured with TFAs] of zero"—there is little concern over the possibility that we were misled. "Not one government agency," wrote Walter Willett, M.D., a Harvard epidemiologist, "has changed its primary [food] guideline to fit the results of the 1990s scientific findings which demonstrate that total fat, including saturated fat, has no relation to heart disease, except for TFAs." "Scandalous," he adds.

Chapter Six

Why the Cover-up?

The truth about the dangers of manufactured TFAs eventually became known to the companies who specialized in manufacturing hydrogenated oils, much as the cancer-causing dangers of cigarette smoking eventually became known to tobacco companies. The TFA cover-up ranks among the big clandestine conspiracies of our corporate culture.

Beginning in 1991 with the publication of major medical outcomes on the risks of TFAs from Harvard University, the fight to keep TFAs off food labels was, as a Food and Drug Administration source told me in a telephone interview in October 2001, "being fought at primarily an economic level."

Economic considerations, not concern for the health of the consumer, frequently propel marketing decisions. Alerting consumers to the dangers of the existence of killer TFAs in foods would have an immediate negative effect on the financial structure of the hydrogenation industry, the packaged-food industry, and the edible oil industry—not the least of which would be the cost of redesigning labels and packages and inventing and testing new recipes.

Now that the FDA has finally mandated that TFAs be listed on food labels by the year 2006, manufacturers will incur inconvenient expenses. But the down side will last only a short time. Like any repair of something gone wrong, the costs will ultimately be absorbed, and the results will make the changes more than worthwhile.

The lethal nature of manufactured TFAs was one of the issues that political and industrial lobbyists were able to keep moving from desk to desk and back again for all those years that the American diet was being saturated with TFAs. Paradigms that become crucial to industry economics—that saturated fat causes heart disease, that statin drugs (which lower LDL cholesterol) prevent heart disease, that hydrogenated oil is a good cooking fat—have proponents with hardworking lobbies in place. Industry also offers incentives to professionals who help their cause.

An example: after the National Cholesterol Education Program of the National Heart, Lung, and Blood Institute announced its 2001 protocol, which included the suggestion that all Americans with elevated LDL (the cholesterol that damages) be prescribed statin drugs, it was revealed that the board of decision-makers had all received honoraria for previous research projects from the drug companies that manufacture statin drugs. In addition, the protocol denounced saturated fats and suggested that people with high cholesterol eliminate butter from their diets and use the newly developed stanol/sterol fat spread substitutes that look and taste like margarine.

Since the advisory recommended foods—the spreads—I called Dr. James Cleeman, coordinator of the program, to ask if any of its board members, advisers, and guest physicians had also received honoraria from any of the food-manufacturing companies that stood to benefit from the manufacture of the stanol/stero spreads. Dr. Cleeman replied that "to ask that question of the board members would be insulting and humiliating to them, as they had already answered routine questions regarding drug company honoraria and would have included food-industry honoraria as a matter of course."

Not necessarily, I thought.

Health

Chapter Seven

Heart Disease and TFAs

Hydrogenated corn and safflower oil margarines; vegetable shortenings, such as Crisco or Spry; corn and safflower oil for frying; white meat of chicken; and artificial eggs made with hydrogenated vegetable oils: These became the standards of the American crusade for better health in the 1950s. For some, they remain the ideal.

Heart disease remains an epidemic. Although consumption of butter and red meat declined in the fifties, sixties, seventies, and eighties, the mortality figures for heart attack did not improve at all.

In the 1950s our population was roughly 175 million. Today we are nearly 300 million. Today 500,000 people die of coronary artery disease each year, the same number as died of coronary disease in the 1950s. It is true that the number of deaths per capita has gone down, but bear in mind that today millions of Americans are saved from coronary deaths each year only by such sophisticated medical interventions as bypass surgery, balloon catherization, and a medicine cabinet stocked with prescription drugs.

It's clear that heart disease has not been cured, that the American diet plan of the last fifty years was not the answer. Cardiovascular disease still kills more Americans than the next seven causes of death combined, including all kinds of cancer.

In 2001, the Centers for Disease Control and the American Heart Association released the following daunting figures:

- 60,800,000 Americans have one or more types of cardiovascular disease.
- 12,600,000 Americans have coronary artery disease—heart attack or chest pain with shortness of breath.
- There are at least 5,400,000 procedures for heart disease performed each year in the United States.
- The cost of cardiovascular disease and stroke in the United States in 2001 was estimated at almost $300 billion.
- Heart disease is no longer a disease only of adults; heart disease can now begin in childhood.

HEART DISEASE RISES IN YOUNG PEOPLE was the headline of an article in the *New York Times* in March 13, 2001. Sudden cardiac death in fifteen- to thirty-four-year-olds in the United States has been rising each year, the article reported. In 1996, 3,000 young people died of sudden cardiac death, 21 percent of the deaths occurring before the age of twenty-four. One of the causes of death was deterioration of the heart muscle, reported the lead author of the study, Dr. Zhi-Jie Zheng, an epidemiologist at the Centers for Disease Control.

Studies Connecting Heart Disease to TFAs

Over the past twenty years, Harvard University has spent over $100 million on three studies: The Nurses' Health Study, the Health Professionals Follow-Up Study, and the Nurses' Health Study II. The results of these studies demonstrate clearly that the risk of cardiovascular disease correlates to the consumption of TFAs: that the people who eat food with the most partially hydrogenated vegetable oils are those most likely to develop heart disease.

Drs. Walter Willett and Alberto Ascherio and their colleagues at the Harvard University School of Public Health estimate that the elimination of partially hydrogenated vegetable oils from the American diet would prevent at least thirty thousand deaths from heart disease and possibly as many as 100,000 additional related vascular deaths *every year.* Moreover, the many millions more who are living with heart disease or developing the disease but don't know it may also have it halted.

The FDA itself has estimated that by removing all TFAs from just margarine and only 3 percent from baked items, more than 17,000 heart attacks and more than 5,000 deaths could be prevented every year. This statement doesn't even consider what miraculous results we might have if other TFA-laden foods, like frozen foods, chips, nondairy creamers, or candy were made TFA-free.

In 2002, the American Heart Association Scientific Conference on Dietary Fatty Acids and Cardiovascular Health announced: "Based on a large body of evidence it is apparent that the optimal diet for reducing the risk of chronic disease is one in which . . . trans fatty acids [TFAs] from manufactured fats are virtually eliminated" and "Trans fatty acids [TFAs] are strong predictors of increased coronary risk compared with saturated fat. . . ."

Chapter Eight

What We Know About TFAs and Health

Manufactured TFAs are a unique danger to humans—a danger that didn't exist until the turn of the last century, when hydrogenation of vegetable oils became possible. These chemically manufactured artificial fatty acids cannot be metabolized by humans.

Manufactured TFAs fool your cells. They masquerade as natural fatty acids, so instead of rejecting TFAs as aliens, cell membranes accept them. TFAs hamper your body's ability to run like the finely tuned machine it is. They have been referred to as "newfangled fats," "artificial fats," and "funny fats" by science writers and medical researchers. But there's nothing funny about them—although the presence of TFAs in our food does make a joke out of any assumption that we are being cared for by the Surgeon General's office.

This short chapter describes what is being documented as the harmful consequences of TFAs, to the heart and circulatory system. Medical and scientific investigators continue to look into the effect of TFAs in other medical areas, including type 2 diabetes (the kind of diabetes increasing numbers of young children and teenagers are diagnosed with), various cancers, and Syndrome X (a disease characterized by insulin resistance, obesity, especially around the belly, elevated cholesterol, and high blood pressure).

Researchers are asking and investigating:

- If TFAs may be why more children are having heart attacks than ever before;
- If there is a connection between TFAs and the little-discussed epidemic of infertility in young and middle-aged married couples;
- Whether and how impaired cellular membranes precipitate cancers;
- What role TFAs have in the raging obesity and type-2 diabetes epidemics in this country;
- How TFAs specifically affect the strength and flexibility of coronary arteries.

Though we do not have answers to these questions, we already know that TFAs don't belong in our food or bodies. Here's what has been documented so far:

1. Cell design allows for normal bodily function. Cells cannot distinguish between real fat and manufactured TFAs. When you eat the manufactured TFAs in a handful of Ritz crackers, its fatty-acid molecules are absorbed into your cells, filling the space that healthy fats ordinarily occupy. Once the artificial fat is in place, the cell cannot reject it, and once the integrity of the cell membrane is compromised, normal cell behavior is compromised and the cell's metabolism is altered. This cellular confusion disrupts vital biological exchanges between cells.

2. Manufactured TFAs raise the damaging LDL cholesterol in your blood and lower the "good" HDL cholesterol, the opposite of what is optimal for heart health. Studies

such as the Nurses Health Study I and II and the Health Professionals Follow-up Study, Harvard School of Public Health, have been providing consistent evidence that the consumption of trans fatty acids increases the risk of coronary heart disease. "When ingredients with no known nutritional benefit are added to foods," says Alberto Ascherio, M.D., "a low threshold for evidence of harm should be adopted, and it should be the responsibility of food manufacturers to show their products are safe."

3. TFAs may upset the balance of arterial cell behavior and lead to soft, weak, and stiffened arteries. Healthy arteries are strong and flexible. Soft, weakened arteries are more susceptible to arterial lesions and consequent heart disease.

Arteries have three layers. The innermost endothelium layer comes into direct contact with blood flowing through the vessel. When an arterial lesion in the endothelium layer is formed (caused by a large range of events that include an excess of carbon monoxide in the blood from cigarette smoking, TFAs, and clotted or thickened blood), cholesterol, a natural healer, rushes in to repair the damage. Because of the weakness of the artery or its sabotage by alien substances, lesions frequently reoccur. Once again cholesterol rushes to the site to make repairs. Successive repairs cause a narrowing of the artery: Layer after layer of cholesterol is built up.

This cholesterol buildup is known as plaque. If a plaque layer gets too thick, it can cause a blockage in the artery that prevents blood from getting to the heart. Plaque can also separate from the arterial wall, resulting in a "blood clot." Heart attacks occur from blockages in the artery and from blood clots.

Endothelial damage is one of the first steps in the sequence of blood vessel damage leading to coronary heart disease.

4. TFAs, like many substances—alcohol, drugs (recreational & prescription), carbon monoxide from cigarette smoke, pesticides—pass from a pregnant woman's placenta to her unborn child. The unborn child's metabolism is adversely affected by TFAs in proportion to the amount consumed by its mother.

5. Lactating mothers who consume substantial amounts of manufactured TFAs have less cream in their breast milk, since TFAs can lodge in cellular spaces normally reserved for fatty acids. This cream, a special fat, is essential for maximum brain development of an infant.

6. Diets high in manufactured TFAs correlate with the risk of Type 2 diabetes. The continuing Nurses' Health Study I and II and the Health Professionals Follow-up Study conducted by the Harvard School of Public Health—a cohort of over 300,000 individuals (approximately 10,000 of whom have developed Type 2 diabetes)—found that nurses (mostly women) whose diet had the most TFAs had a distinctly higher risk of developing Type 2 diabetes. According to the study results, by controlling important behavioral risk factors—engaging in at least moderate exercise, avoiding excess weight gain, avoiding partially hydrogenated fats, and eating whole grain carbohydrates—the risk of developing Type 2 diabetes can be greatly ameliorated. Type 2 diabetes, previously only the province of adults, is now also a disease of teens and preteens in the United States, with children as young as eight (although that is rare) becoming its victims. "In 1992 most pediatric endocrinologists . . . would have said that about 2 to 4

percent of their patients with diabetes had Type 2," said Francine Kaufman, M.D., a professor at the University of Southern California. "Now the data is somewhere between 8 and 40 percent . . ."*

With Type 2 diabetes, the body makes insufficient insulin to overcome shortcomings in the metabolism of glucose. As a result, too much glucose ends up in the bloodstream, which can damage the circulatory and nervous systems as well as major organs such as the heart and eyes. (In Type 1, or juvenile, diabetes the body's *own* defense system attacks and kills insulin-producing cells, which are imperative for storing and using glucose. Most children and adults who have Type 1 diabetes must use insulin to stay alive.) The major increase in Type 2 diabetes, both in children and adults, results from the surge of obesity over the last twenty years—not only in this country, but in Europe as well. Obesity, when not caused by a genetic imbalance, is the result of a high-calorie diet consisting of a preponderance of high-fat (chips, fries, donuts, pizzas), white flour–based (cookies, crackers, hamburger and frankfurter rolls, cakes), and high-sugar foods (colas, sweetened fruit juice drinks, sugared cereals, ice cream); very few whole grains, fruits, and vegetables; and a sedentary lifestyle most certainly encouraged by the electronic marketplace. Notice that the high-calorie foods listed above usually have partially hydrogenated vegetable oils as their primary fat. Obesity kills 300,000 people each year and costs $117 billion in medical bills and lost productivity, reported Denise Grady in *The New*

---

* "As Diabetes Strikes Younger, Children Get Lessons in Self Defense," Randi Hutter Epstein, *The New York Times,* February 20, 2001.

WHAT WE KNOW ABOUT TFAs AND HEALTH   51

York Times. It is on the World Health Organization's list of major global health risks.*

7. TFAs inhibit the absorption of vitamin K into bones. Vitamin K is essential for healthy bone formation and strength.

(Source material for these results can be found in Appendix C.)

If your body has not yet shown signs of noticeable heart disease, hormonal abnormalities, or insulin resistance, that's terrific—but remember, TFAs begin a cumulative chain of silent destruction. If you are one of the 60 million Americans with cardiovascular disease, by eliminating TFAs you can help stop or slow its downward spiral.

Your cells need not be forever compromised by the glut of TFAs they have been fed. After you stop eating foods that contain them, TFAs will gradually disappear from your cells, and the spaces in your cells that were filled with TFAs will gradually be replaced by healthy fatty acids. Even if there is residual damage from your past eating, eliminating TFAs will at least arrest its progression.

You can start that process today.

---

* "What Should We Eat?" Denise Grady, *The New York Times,* November 11, 2003.

PART TWO

Eliminating TFAs from Your Home and Diet

Now that the danger of TFAs is official, you have choices to make about how you feed your family. Your grocery shopping is now a health decision: What you make available for you and your children to dine or snack on affects both your and their well-being. In fact, it would not be going too far to say that what you buy to eat at home and what you eat out at restaurants and fastfood places may be matters of life and death.

But changing your diet doesn't have to be a hardship. In part 2, you will learn how to spot the hidden killer in our foods and to reconsider how you shop and restock your kitchen. I will give you suggestions for improving your food choices and preparing delicious, healthy alternatives to foods containing TFAs. The simple fact is that TFAs are not necessary for good eating; they never have been and they never will be.

Chapter Nine

Reading and Understanding Labels

On July 9, 2003, the FDA announced that it will require food processors to follow a new protocol for labeling all packaged food. As now, labels will continue to list other important nutrients contained in each package, and the ingredients list will still indicate partially hydrogenated vegetable oil.

This new FDA requirement gives manufacturers until January 1, 2006, to change the dietary information on their packaging. The regulation on TFAs also requires that ingredient lists be available to customers in bakeries, fast-food stops, restaurants, take-out shops, airport food stands, food carts, zoo and museum cafés, and hospital cafeterias. Lists have been, in fact, a requirement since the very first labeling laws went into effect in 1991, but only rarely do consumers ask for them, and only rarely do food establishments make those lists easily available. We can only wait to see how this component of the regulation will be adhered to. Chains like Starbucks and McDonald's usually do have the bad news available, but not always.

Knowing what you know now, you must wonder why the FDA doesn't require manufacturers to entirely eliminate partially hydrogenated vegetable oils from manufactured food.

Because the food and oil industries have enormous influence on policy-making government agencies like the FDA. After all, nicotine is still in cigarettes. The history of the battle for mandated packaged food labeling—what to include, what to list separately, who claims what about what fat, and especially the issue of combining different fats into one category—is cluttered with accusations and anger.

The wars were between the edible (vegetable) oil consortiums, promoting the theory that saturated (animal) fats cause heart disease and vegetable oil products don't, and the beef and dairy industries, trying to regain some of the market they lost to hydrogenated vegetable oils, chicken, and artificial eggs. The oil and antisaturated-fat lobbyists were and are retained by specific industries with obvious financial interests. Aside from these, the soybean, corn, and other oil-producing industries have high stakes in this battle as well. So do many drug companies, providing honoraria to research projects and to individuals who sit on committees making high-level policy decisions. Drug companies also offer free or low-fee continuing-education credits to physicians. The subsidized continuing-education courses and other perks designed to lull responsive physicians to write more prescriptions of the sponsor's products are an ever-increasing issue. Physicians medicate our nation. Our health is determined, it seems, not by the moral responsibility of industry—including many physicians—but by its power.

We will have to act for ourselves until the government bans TFAs from food, as it has banned the use of DDT on our crops. You don't have to wait until 2006 for the labeling law to go into effect. Here's how you can become a TFA spotter now.

Look for the Magic Words: Partially Hydrogenated Vegetable Oils

At the moment, the only way you can tell if there are manufactured TFAs in food is by scrupulously scanning the ingredient list (*not* the Nutrition Facts) on the side, back, or bottom of the package. If you see the words "partially hydrogenated" on the ingredient list, you know the food contains TFAs. It's as simple and straightforward as that.

The partially hydrogenated oils may be soybean, coconut, canola, palm, cottonseed, corn, or safflower. Most hydrogenated oil is soybean, but which one doesn't matter. One hydrogenated oil is *not* better than another, no matter what you have heard or a friend or colleague has told you. All hydrogenated vegetable oils are equally harmful to your health— they all contain the killer molecule TFAs.

The terms mono hydrogenated margarine, vegetable shortening, and simply shortening all disguise the fact that the product contains partially hydrogenated oils and therefore manufactured TFAs. This is true even if the front of the package claims "no fats" or "no trans fatty acids."

How is this possible? Because a product that has less than a half a gram (0.5) of TFAs in a serving (the size of a serving is stated on the package) is permitted by the FDA to be advertised as TFA-free. (The new labeling requirements do not change this.) Take Benecol, for instance, a soft-spread substitute for margarine or butter that is advertised as the "good-for-your-heart" spread. Benecol contains a half gram of TFA per serving, a serving being 1½ teaspoons. Recommendations for this product, which is endorsed by physicians and advocated by the National Education Cholesterol Program, are to use it liberally, at least three times a day.

Let's say the consumer uses Benecol on his morning toast (lots of it, even, because the package claims it is *good* for your heart). Maybe he uses it in his sandwich at lunch and on his baked potato and vegetables at dinner. And say he uses two teaspoons (who measures?) of the spread on each item. This Benecol customer has consumed about two grams of TFA by the end of the day. And the Nurse's Study of Harvard's School of Public Health tells us that consumption of just two to three grams of TFAs daily increases the risk of coronary heart disease by 21 percent.

If our determined consumer uses Benecol three times a day, every day of the week, typical use for this kind of spread, he consumes 14 grams a week in Benecol alone. The same consumer may, in the course of a week, also enjoy a hamburger or two grilled with hydrogenated oils or potatoes fried in them. Perhaps every day he eats a handful of crackers or cookies that have them. You can see that it's easy to consume lots of TFAs. They are, after all, in most of the 49,000* different packaged foods typically offered on our grocery shelves and in most of the fast food we've come to rely on. An average meal from McDonald's, for instance, contains three grams of trans fats.

Now, remind yourself that the Institute of Medicine has warned that there is no safe intake level for these killer molecules.

By reading labels and choosing healthier foods, you can begin right now to eliminate manufactured TFAs from your diet. Check ingredient listings for partially hydrogenated vegetable oils on packages you have stocked in your pantry; if you find any, throw the items away or don't buy them again. When you're at the market, read those labels. If they say "partially hydrogenated vegetable oils," keep moving down the aisle.

---

* Bob Earl, senior director for nutrition policy of the National Food Processors Association, in a phone interview in March 2002.

Nutrition Facts	Amount Per Serving	% Daily Value*	Amount Per Serving	% Daily Value*
	Total Fat 8g	12%	Total Carbohydrate 14g	5%
Serving Size 1 patty (63g)	Saturated Fat 1.5g	8%	Dietary Fiber 1g	8%
Servings Per Container 9	Cholesterol 0mg	0%	Sugars less than 1g	
Calories 130	Sodium 120mg	5%	Protein 1g	
Calories from Fat 70	Potassium 140mg	4%		
	Vitamin A 0% • Vitamin C 4% • Calcium 0% • Iron 0%			

INGREDIENTS: POTATOES, PARTIALLY HYDROGENATED VEGETABLE OIL (SOYBEAN AND/OR CANOLA), S DEXTROSE, DISODIUM DIHYDROGEN PYROPHOSPHATE (TO RETAIN NATURAL COLOR).

Figure 1: Take a close look at label A above. On one part of the information label you see the "Nutrition Facts," various percentages of fat (saturated and mono), sodium, carbohydrates, protein. Now skip to the list of ingredients and look for the words "partially hydrogenated vegetable" (or soybean, canola, coconut, palm, or safflower) oil. This one phrase tells you what you need to know about the presence of TFAs in your package. If you see it, stay away. I do not recommend trying to do the math regarding how much of the various fats you will be eating. My focus in this book is on avoiding any package with the killer trans fatty acids.

Become a Label Detective

Until the FDA insists that partially hydrogenated vegetable oils be totally eliminated from food products (instead of only mandating that the presence of TFAs be listed on packages), one problem will continue to exist. New products with consumer appeal and *with* hydrogenated oils will continue to appear. It may be harder to hide TFAs in products, but this won't keep wily entrepreneurs from inventing labels designed to trick you into buying. That is their job. Your job is to keep reading labels, front and back. It takes only a short time to become a proficient label-reader, and then the chore becomes an act of discovery, especially when you find interesting new foods to bring home—and you will.

Some packaged food companies use labels that deliberately mislead, even though they are within FDA guidelines. No trans fats may really mean "half a gram of trans fats," which, if consumed multiple times daily, is more than a body should be subjected to.

Always question advertising on the front of the box that reads:

Low Cholesterol
No Cholesterol
Trans Free
TFA-Free
or
Fat-Free

These slogans may be camouflaging the truth yet remain within the very loose requirements of the law. Furthermore, many packages have labels that are designed to attract children, featuring familiar characters or graphics from television advertising. These labels tempt children with free gifts and seduce them to be loyal consumers of a particular product. Advertising to children is designed to begin early the process of addicting children to unhealthy foods. Read the ingredients list, not the promotion label. Begin to teach your children label sleuthing. The following labels conceal the presence of TFAs in their products:

INGREDIENTS: ENRICHED FLOUR (WHEAT FLOUR, NIACIN, REDUCED IRON, THIAMINE MONONITR VEGETABLE SHORTENING (PARTIALLY HYDROGENATED SOYBEAN AND/OR COTTONSEED OILS) (SODIUM BICARBONATE, SODIUM ACID PYROPHOSPHATE, MONOCALCIUM PHOSPHATE

Figure 2: As you know now, trans fatty acids can be concealed in a number of different terms. In this ingredient list, you see both "vegetable shortening" and partially hydrogenated oil. Always check for the word "shortening," as well as partially hydrogenated vegetable oil, when scanning labels.

INGREDIENTS: SOURDOUGH FRENCH BREAD, B
THIAMINE MONONITRATE, RIBOFLAVIN, FOLIC
ACID. SPREAD: MARGARINE, ROMANO CHEESE,

Figure 3: On this label, trans fatty acids are in the "margarine."

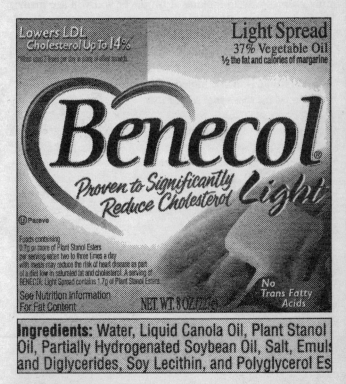

Ingredients: Water, Liquid Canola Oil, Plant Stanol
Oil, Partially Hydrogenated Soybean Oil, Salt, Emuls
and Diglycerides, Soy Lecithin, and Polyglycerol Es

Figure 4: Here is an example of some perfectly legal false advertising. Notice that
the front of the package says, "No Trans Fatty Acids." Now look at the ingredients
list and you will find "Partially Hydrogenated Soybean Oil." That's because the
USDA allows a company to claim "No Trans Fatty Acids" or "No Trans Fats" if their
product contains up to 0.5 grams of TFAs.

Labels on TFA-Free Packaged Foods

There are packaged foods available right now that are totally free of manufactured TFAs, with more manufacturers each month reconsidering their use of partially hydrogenated vegetable oils. But not all are adhering to the idea that none is the only correct way. In looking at products, you will see many misleading come-ons. If the package clearly says on the front "no hydrogenated oils" or "hydrogenated oil free" you can be assured of a TFA-free product. But, as you saw with Benecol above (page 61) the phrase "trans-free" on a package may mean nothing. Don't be fooled by a come-on on the front of a package. *Read those ingredient lists.*

Chapter Ten

Shopping Tips: Searching for What's TFA-Free at the Market

So what can we eat? All fruits and vegetables, fresh meat, fresh chicken, and fresh fish; milk, butter, cheese that is not processed with partially hydrogenated oils, and eggs—these are all natural, all TFA-free. All uncooked grains and pastas are fine, as are raw nuts, dried fruits, and seeds. *Some* tub margarines are okay; read the label. Sugar and spices are TFA-free. So is flour and many breads. Olives and pickles don't have manufactured TFAs (but watch out for that jar of vegetables in oil. Some have them, some don't). And many manufacturers are eschewing partially hydrogenated oils.

If you want to reverse the damage caused by TFAs, you can't afford to wait until 2006, when packaged food labels must be changed. You must stop shopping for products with hydrogenated vegetable oils now. This is something you *can* do.

The marketplace can feed you well. It has been feeding those of us who have known the facts for years. Optimism about the many opportunities around you will get you through the tough beginning. You have a big decision to make. Passivity is comfortable. But now that the danger is official, passivity will be not only an embarrassment but also an injustice to your family.

By now you have the skills to be a careful label reader. As you begin to search for new foods, don't try to do too much too quickly. I recommend selecting one category of food to examine closely on each shopping trip. One day, read the ingredients on the four or five packaged frozen foods you ordinarily purchase. If they are TFA-free, great. If not, check other brands. On another day, check out frozen desserts. Check breads the next time.

Households vary. Some pantries have lots of snack foods, cookies, crackers, and chips, which are frequent TFA-carriers. Instant dinners are popular in other homes. Many of them contain partially hydrogenated vegetable oils. Some families rely more on pastas, rice, and other grains, which are TFA-free, but the same family may unknowingly use sauces that contain TFAs.

Though by no means a complete list of what's in the marketplace, Appendix B (page 133) can help you begin the process of familiarizing yourself with what's TFA-free. Look for those cereals and food bars we've listed, for instance, and jot down other hydrogenated-free cereals and snacks you discover as you shop. This exercise should add only a few minutes to your shopping. It's not necessary to make decisions about buying if you don't have the time. This is a learning experience, and the market is your classroom.

Remember: you want to read the ingredients list, not the advertising label or the Nutrition Facts, to spot partially hydrogenated vegetable oil. And as you shop, remind yourself that your don't-buy list includes the ingredients "margarine," "vegetable shortening," "shortening," and "hardened vegetable oil," all generics for "partially hydrogenated vegetable oils."

A few tips to get you started:

- Do not go shopping with a stomach aching for lunch. Judgment is often impaired by the need for speed;

- Shop with a friend or partner who's also on a TFA-free mission. It's much more fun;
- Wear comfortable shoes and carry a sweater for those freezing refrigerated aisles.

Also carry with you:

- A copy of this book (or take out Appendix B, page 133);
- Reading glasses for the small print on packages;
- Pen and notebook;
- Your shopping list;
- A list of your family's favorite prepared foods.

Now, let's go shopping.

No, You Don't Have to Give Up Those Jelly Bellies

If Skippy's smooth peanut butter (heavy on hydrogenation) is your nine-year-old's favorite food, look for a creamy peanut butter without hydrogenated oils to replace it. Sitting next to the partially hydrogenated Skippy and Jif, you may find two popular unhydrogenated brands: Laura Scudder's (some) and Adams. Both come in crunchy or smooth. Your children may find them too different the first few times they try them, but in no time at all they'll believe it's the best peanut butter they ever tasted.*

If your personal favorite is a Carr's cracker, you'll be disap-

---

* Peanuts are an especially healthy food, containing high levels of oleic acid, a very good fatty acid. Two new "heart-healthy" varieties developed by the Department of Agriculture will be on store shelves (and in peanut butters) in 2004. Some people are allergic to peanuts so the department has recently begun breeding a hypoallergenic variety. Until these are readily available, if you have an allergic family member, try cashew or almond butters. The rest of the family may convert; they're terrific, if also more expensive.

pointed to discover that all of Carr's cracker products are full of TFAs. In the cracker aisle, look for one of the great substitutes, Courtney's Fine English Water Crackers: similar packaging, superior taste, no TFAs. You'll see other brands you never noticed before and old brands you may not have tried, like Ak-Mak crackers or the no-fat, no-sugar Saltines (Premium Saltines are made with partially hydrogenated vegetable oil). Jot down the names of any that look interesting and meet your TFA-free criteria and buy a box or two for comparison.

A few shelves away from the crackers are cookies. One of America's most beloved cookies, Oreos, is a TFA-delivery system. Fortunately, Newman's Own Newman-O's (also Ginger-O's and Hint o'Mint-O's) are a delicious substitute. Check the ingredients to satisfy your curiosity. Make a note.

Check the pretzel assortment: Many pretzels do not contain partially hydrogenated vegetable oils. But as with most brands of chips some flavors of a brand of pretzel will have partially hydrogenated oil, a few will not. Don't trust an entire brand line unless the manufacturer states never using partially hydrogenated vegetable oils in its foods. Check Appendix B for varieties made without partially hydrogenated vegetable oils.

In fact, there are lots and lots of crackers, cereals, granolas, candy bars, and soups manufactured without partially hydrogenated vegetable oil, and you'll soon have new favorites of each. You'll be relieved (and rewarded) to find many wonderful choices of breads, chips, pretzels, dips, and biscuit mixes made without partially hydrogenated vegetable oils. Most Hershey's chocolates don't have TFAs, though some do. Nibbles as Jelly Bellies and blue corn chips are TFA-free. Some ice creams don't have them, others do. Amazing, isn't it, how often partially hydrogenated vegetable oils are slipped into our foods?

There will be many shocking surprises as you read the

labels and discover that certain foods you may think of as healthy, like some cereals made by Quaker, Wheat Thins by Nabisco, or various "nutrition" bars, do contain partially hydrogenated vegetable oils and their payload of TFA poison.

Krispy Kreme donuts have them; lots of Safeway bakery products have them; many Entenmann's cakes have them. Look at the large chain markets, like Wal-Mart and Costco; check their baked goods including their breads. In September 2003, I went to Costco and found that its Kirkland brand Apple Pie and Apple Turnovers are made with partially hydrogenated vegetable oils, as was a box of Belgian chocolates. Stocked, too, on that day were special giant-size boxes of Cheese Doritos, Pepperidge Farm Goldfish, Triscuits, and Premium Saltines—all with partially hydrogenated vegetable oils.

Of course, it is easier to walk down the aisle simply tossing foods into your cart. And yes, reading the label takes time. But just think what the difference will be in the quality of the food you feed your family and yourself and, ultimately, in the quality of life you establish for your household.

Developing a New Brand Awareness

Of course it's hard, especially for children, to give up their favorite treats, like Oreos, Wheat Thins, or Snickers. Your understanding will make these battles easier, and it won't take long before you find a cookie that looks and tastes like Nabisco's Fig Newtons (try Newman's Own Fig Newmans), a cracker that's a good substitute for Nabisco's Wheat Thins (Kashi's TLC, which stands for tasty little crackers), and a wonderful chocolate bar to replace Mars's Snickers.

You'll be surprised at how quickly you become accustomed to the brand names and specific products that stand for healthy packaged food and at how quickly your tastes will change to accommodate these new foods. Start by familiarizing yourself with the names of the brands in Appendix B. Begin your own list of foods you discover. Your list will be your personal association with new food discoveries.

Fortunately, along with the fresh fruit, vegetables, meat, and fish, bin food is gradually becoming safe food. Many bin granolas and snacks used to contain partially hydrogenated vegetable oil; fewer do today. Still, reading here is essential. The labels for bulk foods are on the bin cover (or should be). Unless it's organic, these foods may contain partially hydrogenated oils. Dried dates, apricots, walnuts, almonds (and nuts of all kinds), seeds, and grains—if not fried or roasted—are free of hydrogenated oils. But check everything else. It's a habit none of us can afford not to have.

You do not have to dispose of every food item in your cupboard, pantry, refrigerator, and freezer when you learn about the dangers of manufactured TFAs. If you give in to panic, your pantry will be emptied and most of your family's favorite snacks gone—all in a day. Don't do it. There is another way.

You can make a number of imperceptible changes in your kitchen immediately. Try several alternatives. Making food choices among those that are essential to your kitchen is a simple way to begin. Replacing your old hydrogenated favorites with TFA-free food is a project that only has upsides. The familiar tastes of your favorite potato chip or fried onions will be ghosts in no time, as you discover replacements that are truly delicious. And you will feel the confidence of choosing well. I myself have done this. It works.

Looking over a Typical Shopping List

Following is a list of food categories you find in your local market, categories that appear on most people's shopping lists. Some categories are clearly TFA-free, others definitely not.

Fresh Fruits and Vegetables

All fresh fruits and vegetables are TFA-free. If you do the major portion of your shopping in this section of your market, your diet and your family's will be of high quality. I know it's hard to prepare dinner from scratch these days, but as you become more selective and defiantly leave behind manufactured TFAs, your shopping habits will probably incline toward more vegetables and fruits. Using fresh fruits and vegetables doesn't have to be a laborious and time-consuming chore. Vegetables can always be steamed, fruit always cut up.

Fresh Meat, Poultry, and Fish

Never any manufactured TFAs.

Dairy Products

Milk, cottage cheese, cream, cheese, eggs, yogurt: none of these contain manufactured TFAs. But some imitation cheeses locked in heavy plastic packs, as in a snack box, do. Some processed canned milk-based drinks do. Cool Whip does. You have to check your ice cream selections, too, and become familiar with new flavors and brands.

Breads

The bread section is very interesting. You'd think that the much maligned white bread would be a haven for TFAs and any kind of darker bread, especially the denser, chewier ones, would be the healthier choice. But several white breads do not contain hydrogenated oils, and many dark breads do. The only way you can tell is by looking for those magic words in the list of ingredients: partially hydrogenated vegetable oil.

Cereals

Check the ingredient lists for packaged cereals and bin tops for granolas sold in bulk. For long shelf life, many nonorganic bulk granolas have partially hydrogenated vegetable oils, as do many packaged cereals.

Frozen Foods

The frozen food section of your market is filled with TFAs. Such natural foods as chicken, spinach, potatoes, and other meats and vegetables are prepared with sauces and fats containing partially hydrogenated vegetable oils. Not to mention the pizzas, breads, cakes, pot pies, burritos, and cheese and noodle meals that also contain TFAs.

Read those labels!

Crackers and Cookies

This section is a virtual arsenal of hydrogenation, but you will find good TFA-free alternatives. When you begin your exploration and are looking for replacements, some of the cookies and crackers will not have the taste you hoped for. They can be returned. All markets are set up to handle such exchanges and returns; they do not incur the loss. They simply send the product back to the manufacturer.

Bakery Products

Unless labels are posted, you'll have to ask about a market's own baked products. I was at a supermarket recently, checking the ingredients for made-on-the-premises donuts. They were made with a flour mixture containing partially hydrogenated vegetable oils and so were the icings. Most large chains, such as the Publix chain in the southeastern United States, have on-premises bakeries that daily produce breads, pastries, and birthday cakes made with hydrogenated vegetable oils. So, as you have already read, do the house-brand baked goods, including bread, at such discount giants as Costco and Wal-Mart.

Packaged Lunch Meats

These may have added TFAs. Check your labels.

Canned Fish

All TFA-free.

Other Canned and Packaged Foods

Such items as spaghetti sauce and other sauces, soups, beans, chilis, canned pasta, instant pasta and rice dinners, stuffings, and instant potatoes may contain TFAs. Keep checking those ingredients lists.

Mayonnaise and Other Condiments, Like Mustard, Ketchup, Pickles, Relishes, Olives, and Salad Dressings

Though mayonnaise and salad dressing may be very high in fat, I rarely see salad dressings that contain TFAs any more. Condiments packaged in vinegar are always a safe choice; those in oil are questionable. Read the ingredients label. (You can, of course, prepare your own salad dressing easily and inexpensively with olive oil and a squeeze of lemon or lime.)

Nondairy Beverages

Coffee, tea, soft drinks, and juices are all TFA-free, but for health's sake, remember that soft drinks and most "juice" drinks are little more than sugared water.

It Can Be Done

You know that food that is truly TFA-free varies with brand, and their availability depends on where you shop. But I have never been in a market, not even in a small town like Blanding, Utah, where I couldn't find some packaged foods free of hydrogenated oil.

It's true that I have had years of sleuthing experience, and it took more time to be creative in Blanding, but in that one-market town, I was able to bring home a bag of groceries without a manufactured TFA. True, I selected more vegetables and fruits than packaged foods—that is my general way of shopping—but I was also able to buy bread, canned Progresso soup, a cracker type of snack, and a package of sliced turkey breast without nitrates or hydrogenated oil.

Change Is Happening

A growing number of retail food stores are dedicated to not carrying packaged food containing partially hydrogenated vegetable oils. These are customarily stores that promote organic products and healthy eating. They can be small local shops or large chains, such as Wild Oats, Whole Foods, and Trader Joe's (Trader Joe's does, however, carry some products with partially hydrogenated oils. You must check your labels.). Most communities do not yet have dedicated TFA-free markets but more are opening. Check your neighborhood supermarket—Safeway, Gristedes, A&P, Food Emporium, IGA,

Piggly Wiggly, Price Chopper, etc. These stores may not be dedicated to organic or TFA-free food, but you are sure to find a broad selection of safe foods if you're willing to read the labels. There are choices available no matter where you shop; they are sometimes harder to locate amid the hydrogenated inventory, but they're there.

Every day, more food companies, restaurants, and even hospital cafeterias make it known on their packages and menus that their products are truly TFA-free, made without partially hydrogenated vegetable oils. Some food manufacturers have never used and will never use partially hydrogenated vegetable oils in their products. Some food companies that are newer to the marketplace see nutrition-concerned customers as potentially profitable consumers. They share a similar philosophy and have begun to label their TFA-free food "no hydrogenated oils," knowing the important information that phrase holds for the knowledgeable customer.

If you do live in a place where it is difficult to shop TFA-free, speak to the store manager. Some proprietors are unaware of the dangers you are now learning about. Some will be shocked at what they're carrying and will be happy to replace the bad with the good. If you bring a list of possible product choices, it is possible the store will make changes. Consult Appendix B for a quick list of TFA-free products to recommend and a partial list of manufacturers that do not use partially hydrogenated vegetable oils in their recipes. Look for their products, and of course the ones you discover for yourself, to be assured that the food you bring home is safe for your family.

Involving Your Family and Friends in the Search

Letting friends know what you are investigating will get you additional forces in the search for TFA-free foods, as well as an army of helpers uncovering more partially hydrogenated oils. No one wants to be left out of this kind of investigation. Include your children or other family members in the hunt for new foods. Children are usually eager to solve problems, to look for a culprit. They will be active allies.

By becoming an informed consumer, you join an existing community of people all across the United States, in small towns and big cities, who are bringing about a crucial change. They are folks like you and me who are changing their shopping habits, shunning foods with partially hydrogenated vegetable oils, inventing alternatives to family diets, making their voices known in their home towns and their local grocery stores and supermarkets. And they will be happy to have you among them.

Chapter Eleven

What Fats and Oils Are in Your Pantry?

If you are using margarine made with partially hydrogenated vegetable oil or if you are using Crisco or any vegetable shortening that is white, thick, and slippery, discard it. Cooking fats like most margarines and Crisco-like vegetable shortenings used for frying and baking at home or commercially in bakeries and factories are the densest hydrogenated fat available. They have the highest percentage of TFAs and turn what could be a perfectly acceptable apple pie, donut, or fried chicken into food that kills.

Know Your Oils

First let's untangle some terminology. There are three basic kinds of cooking fats: saturated, monounsaturated, and polyunsaturated.

Saturated fat is primarily animal fat, the fat of meats and poultry, the fat of butter and eggs. Based on the prevailing supposition that saturated fat causes arterial sclerosis and death from heart disease, many people have shunned these foods, thinking them unhealthy. Actually, saturated fats have important fatty acids, and in moderation are an important part of diets.

Since all fats have the same number of calories and therefore the same propensity to cause weight gain, foods that are high in saturated fat—such as roasts, chops, chicken with skin, duck, cheese, sausage, whole and low-fat milk (low-fat milk derives 32 percent of its calories from fat)—should be consumed in small portions and not necessarily every day.*

High levels of saturated fats are also in foods prepared with dairy products, such as pastries made with butter and eggs, mayonnaise, quiches (eggs, cheese, and butter), and pizza made with cheese and meat.

Unsaturated fat comes, for the most part, from plants. Unsaturated fats fall into two categories, polyunsaturated and monounsaturated. All plant foods contain both plus small amounts of saturated fat. (Tropical oils—palm and coconut—are highly saturated.)

Monounsaturated fats: Monounsaturated varieties have many beneficial effects for the body, among them keeping arteries free of inflammation. The most familiar monounsaturated oil is olive oil, my favorite. Olive oil is high in oleic fatty

---

* Low-fat milk (2 percent) is a successful camouflage of a high-fat food. The 2 percent refers to the weight of the fat in the milk, not its calories from fat. Most people do not know that an eight-ounce glass of low-fat milk derives 31 to 32 percent of its calories from fat! How do we know this? Each eight-ounce portion of milk has 45 calories from fat (5 grams of fat x 9 calories per gram of fat, as indicated on the milk container). Each eight-ounce portion of milk has 140 total calories. Divide the total calories by the fat calories, and voila, your answer is clear. While the American Academy of Pediatrics recommends that children under two years old not be fed low-fat or non-fat (skim) milk, other family members can benefit from lower-fat milk. If you or your children tend toward chubbiness, this is a simple way to reduce fat intake. Since our normal diet has many fats—fat from eggs, meat, fish, butter, oils, nuts, beans, and grains—eliminating an unnecessary fat source does not deprive the body of needed nutrients. Nonfat milk (and yogurt) have the same calcium as low-fat and full-fat milk and yogurt.

acids, a fatty acid that is good for heart health. Other oils with high oleic levels are sesame, peanut, and avocado.

Polyunsaturated fats: Polyunsaturated vegetable oils (soybean, safflower, corn, sunflower) have been broadly used as cooking oils for the past fifty-plus years. Polyunsaturates are also in the corn and other grains that have become the feed of choice for cattle, pigs, and chickens instead of the grass they once dined on. These large infusions of polyunsaturates as feed have upset the fatty acid balance of our bodies, interfering with cellular function and good health. (See p. 81 for more on polyunsaturated fat.)

As a general rule you want to

- Consume smaller quantities of foods high in saturated fats
- Consume moderate amounts of monounsaturated fats, and
- Eliminate *added* polyunsaturated fats in the form of cooking oils as the American diet already has sufficient polyunsaturated fat.

If You Are Using Butter—Keep It

Ah, butter! The sublime. Unfortunately, because it is saturated fat, butter has gained a reputation for causing elevated cholesterol and consequently heart disease.

Today, the saturated-fat theory is under reexamination. We know that heart disease has *not* abated in the fifty years we've eaten less butter. Today using butter for flavor is in the realm of healthy eating—in moderation, just as with any other fat.

Butter has certain irresistible charms. In our house, we keep sweet butter in the refrigerator. I add it to steamed vegetables, just a teaspoon for four people. The flavor is unmistakable. The tiniest bit of butter can change a scrambled egg—even an egg white—from ordinary to luscious. And stirring a bit of butter into a sauce for chicken or fish can make a simple dish elegant.

When spring radishes are in the market (or use daikon radishes at any time of year—these are the large white Japanese radishes now available in most markets), slice and lightly salt them and enjoy with lightly buttered fresh baked crusty bread.

If You Are Using Peanut Oil—Keep It

Unrefined peanut oil is an excellent frying oil without a strong taste that can be heated to the high temperatures necessary for frying. Peanut oil is never hydrogenated.

If You Are Using Extra-Virgin Olive Oil—Keep It

Extra-virgin olive oil is the best oil in town, for taste and for health. Olive oil's proportions of fatty acids make it an ideal companion for our bodies.

Olive trees have been familiar sights on the green slopes of Tuscany and in Greece and Spain for millenia. The allure of Italian and Spanish imported olive oils destroyed a once-thriving California olive oil industry; by the middle of the twentieth century it had virtually disappeared. Now groves are reappearing in California, covering hillsides on the north coast not far from where I live and becoming second crops at wineries throughout the state. With an expanding worldwide economy favoring healthy foods, olive trees are being planted everywhere the climate encourages their growth. Olive oils are never hydrogenated.

The best quality olive oil, and consequently the best for

your body, is extra-virgin. In making extra-virgin oil, olives are cold-pressed using stone rollers moving over granite slabs to extract the olive paste. The modern process mimics to some degree the ancient way of processing olive oil, which employed large stone crushers of various designs, frequently turned by yoked farm animals, sometimes, in Roman provinces, by slaves. The oil obtained by the first pressing, after the pits were removed, was the finest—equivalent to what we call extra-virgin today. The quality of the oil diminishes with each pressing, as does the market value.

As the industry expands, more efficient ultramodern machinery is challenging the romance of stone and granite. But as long as the crushing is done at low heat, the integrity of the fatty acids in the olives and the many natural and good-for-you preservatives in the oil are guaranteed. Make sure to look for a label that says extra-virgin; it guarantees the best processing available.

Because of the cool processing and its high percentage of natural preservatives, olive oil, if stored in a cool, dark place, is unlikely to become rancid.

Purchasing and Caring for Olive Oil

Extra-virgin olive oil at any price can be delicious. You don't have to buy the very high priced, extravagantly bottled brands. Look for extra-virgin olive oil packaged in its country of origin. This tells you that the time between production, transport to the bottling facility, and bottling itself was not excessive and that therefore there was less opportunity for spoilage.

If the price is right, buy your oil in dark-colored bottles, which protects the oil from light. Buy half-liter bottles unless you have a large family and use it frequently. Once the bottle is opened and the oil is exposed to air, spoilage begins, although it proceeds very slowly. This can't be helped, but it can be retarded. Close the bottle after using and keep it stored in a cool, dark place, never on a counter or on a sunny windowsill. Store the oil in a cooler rather than warmer place—away from the stove is best and not near the heat. Air, light, and warmth encourage spoilage of all oils. Refrigerating olive oil doesn't work for daily use: It solidifies, turns grayish, and is not easy to use for several hours after it is removed. But storing it there when you are on a lengthy vacation is a good idea, as is dividing a bottle in half and keeping half in the refrigerator, the other in the pantry.

Cooking with Olive Oil

The best way to use olive oil, in addition to dressing salads and for cold foods, to retain its extraordinary nutritional benefits is to add it *after* cooking. This is because heat breaks down the molecular configuration of oil. So steam your vegetables, then add olive oil to them. Bake your fish after wiping it lightly with oil; and add more when you serve it, if desired. Steam your rice, then add the oil. If you are cooking onions, mushrooms, shallots, celery, or carrots, sauté them in a little water then add the oil after cooking. Drizzle olive oil over grilled tomatoes or steamed mussels after cooking.

Of course, there are times when heated olive oil is needed for what you are cooking—for example, browning chicken or fish, sautéing carrots or cauliflower, or cooking potatoes to a certain crispness.

If You Are Using Polyunsaturated Oils Such As Corn Oil or Safflower Oil, Use Them Rarely or Not at All

Bottled polyunsaturated vegetable oils for cooking (corn, safflower, soy) are not hydrogenated, but they are refined (cleaned with detergents). The use of polyunsaturated oil products for cooking boomed by the 1960s, when medical research strongly suggested that the epidemic of heart disease in America was caused by our saturated-fat (meat, butter, eggs, cream) intake. Replace the butter used for cooking, said the American Heart Association, use corn oil for frying, and buy margarine (corn and safflower) for your bread. Powerful special interest groups also helped to keep polyunsaturated cooking oils in our supermarkets.

Now we know that the large-scale manufacturing and marketing of polyunsaturated cooking oils and the widespread use of polyunsaturates—as corn for stockyard feed (animals used to eat grasses that contain omega-3 fatty acids), as the fat of margarine, and as the raw material for hydrogenated oils—has tampered with the exquisite balance of human cellular synthesis. The healthy dietary ratio of one important fatty acid, omega-6, to another important fatty acid, omega-3, should be four to one: four times as many omega-6s as omega-3s. Yet the American diet has 10 to 30 times more omega-6s! Though our bodies cannot manufacture these fatty acids, they are crucial to maintaining our lives. A deficit of omega-3s leaves us with less perception of pain, compromised cell membranes, which can lead to structurally damaged blood vessels, and robs us of a natural blood thinner.* We do not need to add polyunsaturates in the form of cooking oils to our

---

* Artemis Simopoulos, M.D.

diet. If your diet includes assorted vegetables and fruits, beans, whole grains, nuts such as walnuts and butternuts (high sources of omega-3s), fish, poultry, and even pork, using extra-virgin olive oil as your staple oil is perfect.

Eating wisely, watching your intake of processed foods and using olive oil as your most-used household fat will begin to change the ratio of omega-6 to omega-3 in your body.

And a Word About Two Tropical Oils

There is much confusion and dissension about nonhydrogenated coconut and palm oils, both of which have been used for centuries by Asian Pacific cultures. Coconut oil, while highly saturated, has multiple health benefits. Among others, it contains a large amount of a fatty acid called lauric acid, which inhibits arterial inflammation; lauric acid is also a component of breast milk. Nonhydrogenated palm oil (not palm kernel oil or fractionated palm oil) is the cooking fat chosen for most of Newman's Own Organics after a thorough search to find a healthy alternative to hydrogenated oils.

If you are shopping for coconut oil, look for the phrase "expeller-pressed" on the package or bottle. This phrase means that the oils have been extracted without using chemicals or heat. Nonhydrogenated coconut oil is a good choice as a cooking replacement, always better than a polyunsaturated oil. Nonhydrogenated palm oil, while useful in commercial kitchens for baked goods, does not, in my opinion, have a flavor that makes it kitchen-friendly.

Chapter Twelve

Ideas for the TFA-Free (and Even Lower-Fat) Kitchen

If you are the family cook, you have prerogatives in the kitchen. You can use olive oil or butter instead of margarine. You can throw out your Crisco and fry with peanut oil, a bland-tasting oil with healthy fatty acids and a higher smoke point than other oils (can be heated to a higher temperature before it smokes or burns). No one will even know you've made changes.

Following are some ideas for replacing TFA-containing fats:

- When you fry chicken, chops, fritters, and potatoes, use unrefined peanut oil. To maintain weight and general good health, fried foods, cakes, and cookies should be choices only on rare occasions rather than for everyday eating; they fill you with fat and sugar calories that leave less room for fruits and vegetables, whole grains and fresh meat, chicken, fish, and wholesome dairy products. If you think of fried food and sweet foods as treats, not as daily necessities, your body will soon begin to show the effects of this change.

- If you do bake pies and cookies, replace Crisco or vegetable shortening with butter.
- Replace your TFA-loaded margarine with butter or olive oil, the fats that humans have been using since agriculture and domestic animals replaced the hunter-gatherer tradition. Some new tub margarines are TFA-free. But check carefully: even if the label on the front of the box says, "trans fat–free" or "cholesterol-free," you know now that monitoring the ingredient list on the back of the box is essential. You may be looking at a product that falls within the FDA's allowable half gram (0.5) of TFAs per serving, which lets a food manufacturer claim there is none in its product.

  Ethics are sometimes neglected in marketing decisions. You will know the truth about a food product if you see the words "partially hydrogenated vegetable oil" in the ingredient listing no matter how emphatically the front of the package says it is TFA-free. Playing detective may not be what you had in mind as part of shopping, but it's critical, the only way to keep your family safe from ingredients that kill.
- Use butter or olive oil sparingly; small amounts will add the flavor you are after. The truth is that no fat, olive oil included, is good for you if you pour or glop it on your food.
- If you're used to sautéing foods in margarine, substitute olive oil or use half butter, half olive oil. Keeping in mind that we are a nation of folks who tend to eat more fat (and sugar) than is good for us, if you already sauté in olive oil or butter, consider reducing the amount you use by half. Most of us use much more fat for cooking than is necessary, and recipes, especially newspaper recipes, almost always suggest using larger amounts of fat than the cooking warrants. Soon it becomes a habit

to overuse these ingredients. When you use olive oil for cooking, don't pour it; measure it by the teaspoon; you can always add more. (Other ways of using olive oil is to pour some into a spray bottle and spray it on the bottom of your pan or apply it with a pastry or small paint brush.)

Here are some general, lower-fat cooking suggestions:

- Use a nonstick pan for cooking vegetables, potatoes, chicken breasts, prawns, or small flat fish. You need far less oil or butter for your cooking, and the pans are easy to clean. My favorite nonstick pans are made by Wearever. Their Lincoln CeramiGuard fry pans are made of heavyweight aluminum and come with a rubber sleeve to keep the handles cool. They are widely available in different sizes, are modestly priced, and are the pan of choice in many restaurants.
- Though dairy products are TFA-free, consider a lower-fat version of the milk, yogurt, or cottage cheese you ordinarily use. (See footnote on page 76.)
- Use half as much meat as you usually use in stews and twice the amount of vegetables.
- Prepare stews the day before you serve them and chill the sauce separately. The fat will solidify on top, and you can easily skim it off and discard it.
- Delete two of your family's traditional high-fat meals each week, substituting a simple-to-prepare lower-fat meal with less meat and more vegetables and grains.
- Instead of drowning a salad in dressing, squeeze half a small lemon or lime into a bowl, add Kosher salt and pepper to taste, mixing well to dissolve the salt, then simply whisk in a tablespoon of olive oil. Or, as they do occasionally in Italy, use just olive oil and salt & pepper.

You can also add fresh chopped tomatoes and herbs for additional flavors.

- Delete half your family's high-fat desserts, substituting fresh fruit. Fresh fruit slices with slivered or chopped nuts, candied ginger, dried apricots, or dates make great desserts.

- Choose breads that are whole or mostly whole grain and free of fats and sugars. There are many of these in the supermarket. If you live near a bakery that doesn't use hydrogenated vegetable oils, try its fresh bread.

- When you serve cheese as a snack or in a sandwich, serve it with vegetables, like tomatoes, cucumbers, celery, and lettuce. You will reduce the amount of cheese you eat (a high-fat food) and add new flavors to your sandwich or snack.

- Introduce new snacks into your house to begin the conversion from high-fat, TFA-saturated foods to healthy alternatives. Keep vegetable snacks high on your list. (See snacks on page 137.)

- Make omelets with half the number of yolks you usually use and twice the whites. You will hardly notice the difference. Since the fat of the egg is in the yolk, you will be eating less fat.

- When using cheese in a main dish, use it as a condiment rather than as a significant ingredient.

- You can also use meat and poultry as condiments: for instance, two or three chicken breast halves, sliced and tossed in a rice and mushroom casserole for six.

- Remove the skin from chicken or turkey breasts. Skin *doubles* the calories of the poultry and should be considered as treat food.

- When you brown ground meat, drain it on paper towel to absorb most of the fat before you add it to the rest of the ingredients.

- Canned or aseptically packaged nonfat chicken, beef, and vegetable broths are invaluable cooking staples. Use them in soups, sauces, stews, as an afternoon snack, or make a quick soup with cut up vegetables. As vegetables cook in scant amounts of broth or water—often called "water sautéing"—they soften and brown as if you were using oil. (You can always add a teaspoon of olive oil or butter halfway through the cooking or after the vegetables are done for taste.) "Sautéing" this way will require you to add liquid by the tablespoon until the vegetables are cooked.

Changing Your Children's Lunch Habits— Instantly

Foods without TFAs don't have to torture or embarrass your children. You can provide them a lower fat, TFA-free lunch that they'll hardly notice is different, especially if you introduce these changes slowly and without making the changes, as they would say, "bizarre."

For instance:

- Most sandwich spreads (mayonnaise and mustard) are TFA-free. Mayonnaise is a high-fat spread, but for many people it's an essential ingredient. Take a chance and halve the amount you use.
- Replace cookies and other packaged desserts with ones that do not contain partially hydrogenated oils. Then start a new custom of alternating those TFA-free cookies or cakes with dried or fresh fruits or nuts and fruit. You know your children, and only you know how rapidly you can make changes.
- Substitute homemade trail mixes for candy.

- Substitute TFA-free chips or pretzels for ones made with hydrogenated oils.
- Use bread that contains no hydrogenated oils.
- Use peanut butters made without partially hydrogenated oils. Add apple or vegetable slices to peanut butter sandwiches. Peanut butter is a very healthy food if your child is not allergic to peanuts. It's great at breakfast with orange or apple slices or at lunch with cucumber or celery in a sandwich.

The High Price of Cheap Food—Snacks

Americans are snackers. Much of what we snack on is packaged foods. And most packaged foods contain the manufactured killer TFAs, the fat we don't want to eat. Until food manufacturers climb on the TFA-free bandwagon, we really must take a careful look at what we nibble on in the course of the day and what kind of snacks we keep at home for both adults and children.

You will be pleasantly surprised at the good and growing variety of chips, dips, crackers, cookies, candy, popcorn, pretzels, and pizzas that are TFA-free. So, you may think, terrific!

However, these kinds of foods, largely made from simple carbohydrates (sweeteners and white flour) can eventually skew your and your children's nutritional balance and health, especially when snacks substitute for meals or become a major part of the diet. Meal-size snacking defeats nutritional balance, leaves no stomach room for nutritious foods, such as cooked vegetables and salads, and makes sitting at the dinner table a chore for children who snacked the afternoon away. Processed snack food has become a major source of daily calories—for them and for us.

Snacks should be food bites to see you through a time

when your stomach is rumbling or, as Dr. Walter Willett suggests, something small to "spoil your dinner," to keep you from eating overlarge meals. For me, a few walnuts and an apple will do it, or a shredded cabbage salad, or a dried fig and an ounce-size chunk of cheese. For hungry children who would make faces at cabbage or figs, make a mixture of a nut butter whipped with plain nonfat yogurt. Slice apples or carrots to dip into it. Chips, you'll discover, are not necessary.

Cut-up fruit always seems to tempt both children and adults. Bowls of cut-up fruit at a child's eye level in the fridge were a grand success in our kitchen when our children were growing up.

Changing what you think of as snacks is one of the big challenges to the nutrition-conscious consumer. Snacks from the following list will dramatically change the quality and balance of your diet. By all means, add to it as you discover new, appealing ones.

Olives
Walnuts (raw)
Almonds (raw)
Sunflower seeds (raw)
Green peas (fresh or frozen)
Red radishes or sliced daikon radish
Peanuts
Peanut butter (or any nut butter) mixed with nonfat plain
    yogurt and raw vegetable slices for dipping
Homemade baked potato skins with salsa or freshly
    chopped vegetables
Nonfat plain yogurt with raisins or cut-up fruit
Dry-roasted soy nuts
Dry-roasted or canned garbanzos (chickpeas)
Sliced raw vegetables and fruits
Dried fruit; e.g., apricots, figs, raisins, plums (prunes),

berries, apples, pears, peaches, mango, banana, pineapple

I also like the following fruit combinations for dessert:

Dried figs and walnuts
Dates stuffed with almonds
Sliced summer fruit with currants
A large bowl of fresh cherries for the table accompanied
   by a bowl of almonds
Fresh figs and very thinly sliced sweet Meyer lemon or
   lime
Sliced fuyu persimmon with julienned, sugared, dried
   ginger candy
Fresh plums and strawberries
And always, apples—any way

You might consider preparing your own trail mix for a take-along treat on hikes, for when you go to the movies or attend an athletic event, or to take to work. Nuts, seeds, raisins, and a few semi-sweet chocolate bits make a mix everyone will like.

Drop out of the thirty-billion-dollar-a-year snack-food industry! Encourage good ideas among family members (and friends) for nonsugared foods without processed fat. Have a contest for the most delicious healthy snack a family member makes or finds in the marketplace.

Try New Things

Eliminating TFAs from your body does not mean that you have to eliminate good-tasting food. In fact, it gives you the perfect excuse to expand your diet to include foods that give you more choices, not fewer. The fruits and vegetable aisles of any supermarket provide foods you know are TFA-free; there you can choose whatever you wish. Fruits and vegetables are also important sources of fiber, essential vitamins and other nutrients. Most of us should be eating more of these than we do.

Most of us are familiar with only a limited number of fruits and vegetables and are shy or cautious to try unfamiliar ones. We remain partial to one of a few kinds of potatoes (in Ecuador there are over four hundred different kinds of potato, and while we won't find that variety here, there are at least twenty I can think of as I write), we use only a few kinds of lettuce, a few of apples. You may have seen fennel, bok choy, arugula, chard, and jicama in your market. You may have looked at papayas, apples with strange sounding names, melons from Indonesia, mangoes from Hawaii, fresh figs from California, but not knowing what they taste like or how to use them, even how to eat them, you may have backed away. Many people are not food adventurers. But being bolder will help you find more interesting alternatives in the fruit and vegetable sections.

Talk to supermarket employees in the fruit and vegetable section. If you want to know if the peaches are sweet, ask. They may cut you a slice. If you want to know what jicama or any other fruit or vegetable tastes like, just say so. These employees are there to serve you. They'll tell you all about any fruit and vegetable, where it's from, how to cook and serve it, if they know. I've never met an employee in this section of a grocery store who didn't seem delighted to be asked for information and eager to be of service.

Here are a few simple—perhaps new—vegetable dishes you may want to try in your kitchen:

- For a quick carrot soup, "sauté" carrot sticks in a little broth or salted water until tender. Blend in a blender or food processor. Add a teaspoon of olive oil and finely chopped parsley. You can make a zucchini soup this way as well, perhaps adding a small chopped onion to the cooking broth.

- Add spiced TFA-free tomato sauce or fresh chopped tomatoes to steamed green beans.
- Bake cauliflower pieces with fresh garlic, fresh ginger, salt and pepper. Toss lightly in olive oil before baking.
- Sauté spinach, chard, thinly sliced carrots, shredded cabbage, or other vegetables cut in small pieces, such as cauliflower, broccoli, or young turnips.
- Buy sun-dried tomatoes in bulk and eat them as a snack. Thinly sliced on a peanut butter sandwich, they're an amazing taste treat.
- Toss thin slices of raw fennel into salads, or toss them with sliced mushrooms or celery and olive oil.
- Try bok choy. Cut up two or three regular-size bok choy or six baby ones and "sauté" the pieces in chicken broth. Add a sprinkling of olive oil when the cooking is complete.
- Steam cut-up broccoli in one pan and green beans in another. They're delicious together sprinkled lightly with olive oil and grated parmesan cheese.

If you have never baked fish in foil or parchment packages, you may find it an answer to dirty pans and the sometimes intense odor fish leaves after being cooked indoors. Lay one portion of fish on one half of the foil or paper—the paper should be the width of the foil box and about fifteen inches long—salt and pepper the fish, add a little lemon or lime juice, one tablespoon of white wine or plain water, and a few thin slices of carrot, onion, or both. Fold the paper over the fish and fold down the edges, crimping the paper to seal the packet as you go along. Bake the packages on a cookie sheet in a 350-degree oven for fifteen minutes. Before you open the packet, make a small slit on the side away from you to let the steam escape. Serve the fish with the accumulated sauce. This same method is terrific for chicken breasts. Just lengthen the cooking time to thirty to forty minutes, depending on the size of the breast.

When grilling or broiling steaks or chops or roasting a pork loin, for a different taste, make a dry marinade by grinding two cloves, a star anise, and an herb such as thyme, several peppercorns, and kosher salt. Marinate the meat overnight—or even just an hour or two, if that's all the time you have. Grill, broil, or bake as you usually do.

Here are just a few more of the simple dishes I like to cook for family or friends.

Green and Yellow Pepper Pasta

In a bowl large enough to hold cooked pasta, marinate very thin slices of green and yellow peppers (one pepper per person) in salt, cracked pepper, and 1 tablespoon of olive oil for each person. When the pasta is cooked, add 1 tablespoon of the hot cooking water to the peppers, add the drained pasta, toss, and serve.

Suggested toppings for this dish are finely chopped parsley mixed with grated parmesan cheese or a mixture of parmesan cheese and toasted bread crumbs.

Prawns with Pasta for Lunch

The best lunch! Sitting around a cozy table shelling prawns and licking your fingers is high on my list of a great meal.

Grate 1 teaspoon of lemon zest. Toss unshelled prawns (count on six to eight large-size prawns per person) in kosher salt and red pepper flakes. Poach the prawns in a large frying pan in a quarter-inch of water or white vermouth. Cook for four to five minutes, turning the prawns as they turn pink. Remove from heat, and toss with 1 tablespoon of olive oil for each pound of prawns.

Cook some pasta (a pound feeds four to five). When the pasta is cooked, add the prawns and the lemon zest. Place a bowl in the middle of the table for the prawn shells. A tomato, watercress, and arugula salad is a nice complement to this dish.

Pasta with Chicken or Turkey and Thyme

A great way to use poultry leftovers.
Julienne the leftovers.

For 1 cup of leftovers, make a sauce from 2 tablespoons chicken stock, 1 tablespoon olive oil, kosher salt, pepper, and chopped fresh thyme or a pinch of dried thyme. Pour the sauce over leftover poultry and set aside to marinate while the pasta or rice is cooking. Toss together when the cooking is completed.

Grilled or broiled tomatoes, summer squashes, sautéed chard, are all good accompaniments. A salad of fresh tomatoes, thinly sliced uncooked summer squash, chopped parsley, and lettuce of any kind can be substituted for the cooked vegetables.

Judith's Favorite Pan-Roasted Potatoes

Wipe a frying pan lightly with olive oil.

Boil 4 thinly sliced, unpeeled large potatoes (any kind you like) in salted water until they are barely cooked; depending on the potato, about four minutes. Pat the potatoes dry.

Toss the sliced potatoes with cracked pepper, kosher salt and 2 tablespoons of olive oil.

Arrange the potatoes in the pan so that the slices overlap. Cook for three to four minutes over fairly high heat, moving the pan back and forth across the burner so the potatoes do not burn. Lower the heat to low and cover the pan.

Finish the cooking on low heat for forty-five minutes or until the bottom is browned, uncovering the pan for the last ten minutes. Serve with the brown side up.

Restocking Your Pantry with the Basics

Last, keep a well-stocked pantry, refrigerator, and freezer, filled with TFA-free foods. When you have a good variety of TFA-free staples on hand, you are always ready to create dinner, lunch, or breakfast, round out a fish or meat or rice dish, or save the day with an emergency sandwich or snack.

In my kitchen, I avoid canned and packaged foods that are made with lots of sugar as well, since sugar creeps into everyone's diet. There's no sense in adding unhealthy calories to savory food. And if there's a choice, my preference is always to try a lower-fat item over a higher one. Add your own favorites to the following list of basics:

Pasta, rice, bulgur wheat, barley, and other grains, which are always TFA-free (see chapter 15 for a chart of cooking times for grains)

Dried or canned beans (garbanzo [chickpeas], cannellini, kidney, and black)

A variety of canned soups including nonfat chicken broth and nonfat vegetable broth

Jams (best if fruit, not sugar, is the first ingredient on the label)

Salsas

Tomato juice

Peeled tomatoes in cans or boxes

Tomato pizza sauces

Marinated vegetables (in jars)

Fish packed in tins or cans, such as tuna, salmon, sardines, anchovies

Frozen vegetables, such as corn kernels, peas, spinach, baby lima beans

Bread (whole wheat or other whole grain is best)

Crackers and cookies

Raisins, dried figs, dried peaches, dried apricots, and other dried fruits

Nuts almonds, walnuts, pecans (not fried or cooked), peanuts (raw or dry-roasted if the oil is okay)

Peanut butter or a nut butter, such as almond

Unsweetened applesauce

Sherbets and ice creams in several flavors

Fresh fruit, fresh vegetables, milk, yogurt, cheese, eggs

100% fruit juice Many drinks with "juice" on the label are not fruit. They are primarily sugar or high fructose corn syrup and water

Unprocessed meat, fish, and chicken

Condiments, Sauces, and Flavorings

These qualify as staples, too. All are TFA-free:

Extra-virgin olive oil

Assorted raw seeds (pumpkin, sunflower, sesame)

Olives (try several different types)

Vinegars, plain and mild, like Japanese rice vinegar, or stronger, such as red or white wine, raspberry, tarragon, or balsamic vinegars.

Soy sauce

Worcestershire sauce

Hot sauces and Thai curry pastes

White horseradish (in a jar)

Mustards, dry and prepared

Frozen or refrigerated homemade soup stocks

Dried herbs and spices (be adventurous)

Candied ginger (great sliced and used as a garnish for fruit and yogurt desserts)

Parmesan cheese, and other cheese choices, for grating and nibbling

Store-bought bread crumbs or croutons if you can find them without hydrogenated oils (if not, crush your own from toasted day-old bread)

Dried mushrooms They can be separated into small packages for the freezer. They stay fresher this way and defrost almost immediately.

Capers

Chutneys

Chapter Thirteen

Takeout, Eating Out

In New York City not long ago, I was shopping in an affluent
Upper East Side neighborhood for ingredients to prepare dinner for the friends my husband and I were staying with. When
I set out, I thought it would be a simple task to bring home
some of the delicious looking take-out foods New York is famous for, supplementing them with a salad and homemade
dessert. I was in a neighborhood I'd always considered to
have some of the best food the city offers.

But when I asked at the market, I learned that the oil and fat
used in the preparation of the wonderful looking grilled
chicken breasts and the lamb stew was partially hydrogenated canola oil. The same oil was used for the marinade for
the rotisserie chicken.

While I know personally that there are wonderful New
York stores with prepared foods totally free of hydrogenated
ingredients (Dean & DeLuca and the Vinegar Factory, for instance), I was not at any of those places at five o'clock in the
afternoon on that day. So I changed my plan. I bought an uncooked chicken, dried pasta, broad beans, garlic, and lettuce
to take back to our hosts' apartment to cook supper.

I could do this with good humor because I was on vacation, had no deadline, no business to attend to, no children to

entertain, and I love to cook. But I am well aware that taking prepared food home is something increasingly many people count on, especially in families where both parents work. Make it a point to find out which of the take-out places in your neighborhood use hydrogenated oils in their recipes. This will make the hurried, end-of-the-day shopping less of a chore and certainly leave you in less of a quandary.

Asking for the Ingredients

Every restaurant and take-out eatery, from the muffin vendor on the corner to the delicatessen three blocks away to the gourmet destination, is required to have on hand a list of the ingredients in the prepared foods they sell.

Every neighborhood grocery must have a list, too. Have you ever bought a cellophane-wrapped cookie with no label at all, let alone a list of ingredients? Your grocer may have bought a dozen of those cookies from the manufacturer then rewrapped them in cellophane to sell individually. You'll find wrapped caramels and chocolate-covered cherries, halvah, and baklava, along with other unlabeled foods like hard candies and lollipops near cash registers. They are there for you to buy on impulse, or for your child to wish for. The proprietor has made it easy for you; you can buy as few as one. Most have no ingredients list. Some of these foods may be made with partially hydrogenated vegetable oils, but you cannot tell. Same with the muffins you buy at coffee shops. All are required to have a list of the ingredients used in their pastries somewhere in the store. Ask at the counter: "Can I see the ingredients for the blueberry danish pastry?" Sometimes the list will be there. Often, it will not.

In restaurants you frequent, ask about the bread. Is it made with hydrogenated vegetable oils? If the bread isn't baked there, the restaurant is still required to show you what ingredients it contains.

It helps to remember that a lot of people are profoundly allergic to certain foods. Even the smallest amount of peanuts can be lethal for some people. Many people are lactose-intolerant or allergic to wheat. For these people, asking about ingredients is absolutely necessary. For some it's life or death.

The same is true for you and your family with foods made with hydrogenated oils. The TFAs in partially hydrogenated vegetable oils cause heart disease and play significant roles in obesity and type 2 diabetes; the verdict is still pending on what else. The ingredient hidden in every bite of food made with, fried in, sprinkled on, or spread with partially hydrogenated vegetable oils can kill. For that reason, it's irresponsible *not* to ask what's in the food you're about to buy.

Some Pointers

I'm quite used to asking about ingredients by now, in a genial way. You don't want to be accusatory or demanding. Why would you? The person you ask is most probably innocent, not at all aware of the product he sells. In a bakery I usually ask, "Do you use only butter? Are any of your pies or pastries or breads made with vegetable shortening?"

At my neighborhood take-out counter, I ask what oils they use in their salad dressing, soup, bean salad, chicken salad, mixed vegetables, roasted potatoes, and barbeque chicken. The person at the counter rarely knows. He has to find the manager, who then consults the cook.

Frequently, when you ask for the list of ingredients, people are perfectly happy to oblige; you don't get the impression they at all mind. Increasingly, I find the people who work the serving and cooking end of the food industry to be happy to get the information for you. Occasionally the person I ask will seem irritated, but that's okay. Eating foods with manufactured TFAs is treacherous. And we have a right to know.

Now that the word about the effects of TFAs on health is spreading, you will not be the only one asking for those lists of ingredients. When enough of us ask, change will happen. Next we will ask the coffee shop to offer muffins and cakes made without partially hydrogenated oils. Then we will ask the sandwich shop down the street or the deli counter at the market to carry breads and spreads that don't contain partially hydrogenated oils. This is how change happens. It can easily happen in the small mom-and-pop store in your neighborhood. It can even happen locally in a large chain market. Speak to the manager. She wants you to shop at her market so will be pleased to converse with you.

Just Say No to Fast Food

Fast-food places are important distribution centers for partially hydrogenated vegetable oils. Keep reminding yourself that TFAs hide in dressings and sauces, in sautéed and fried meats, fried chicken, nuggets of all kinds, fried potatoes, sandwiches, cooked vegetables, croutons, taco shells, and burritos. TFAs may also be in muffins and rolls. Sometimes they are in frozen milk shake drinks. They are in almost every nondairy type creamer. If your local fast-food stop does not have a listing for you of the ingredients used in their cooking and preparation, their regional office will. Ask for the phone number. They will mail you an ingredient list.

For the time being, I'm afraid my advice has to be: Do not patronize fast-food places that use hydrogenated vegetable oils, or at least resist the fries, nuggets, muffins, fried chicken, hash browns, taco shells, even sandwiches. About the only thing we can be guaranteed is TFA-free in any of the fast-food places we're accustomed to (McDonalds, Burger King, Taco

Bell, Wendy's, and Arby's) is the salad bar but be sure to check the dressing and skip the croutons.

At Your Favorite Restaurant

At your favorite restaurant, shouldn't you know what's cooking in the kitchen? The folks who run the place might actually appreciate being asked. Ask the cooks, chef, or management if you can glance at the containers for their cooking and frying oil, specifically, the containers the cooking oil arrives in from the distributor. Frequently the cooks or management will not know what you are looking for; they have been convinced by their edible-oil salesperson that the product is good, healthy vegetable oil. This could be the moment of their reeducation.

Many, if not most, luncheonettes, diners, and small local spots deliver TFAs by using hydrogenated oils in salad dressings, to deep-fry, or on the grill to toast frankfurter rolls, cook home fries, and scramble eggs. Ask your local owners to change to plain peanut oil for frying and olive oil for cooking and dressings. If your neighborhood restaurant cooks with margarine, it will usually be the kind made with partially hydrogenated vegetable oils. Explain the downsides of these cooking fats. Walk in with a pad of paper and a copy of this book. Look important. You are—you are saving lives.

And Other Places

Yes. Sigh. Many pizzerias, delicatessens, and Chinese, Thai, Burmese, Caribbean, and kosher restaurants cook with oils or fats (margarine included) loaded with TFAs. Those great Thai soups, Chinese dumplings, chicken satays, and tandoori meats may all have been cooked with hydrogenated oils. Japanese restaurants sometimes use these oils for tempura and stir-frying.

I have a particular fondness for sushi and other Japanese foods. In 1995, when I asked about their cooking oils at my favorite Japanese restaurant, Kirala, in Berkeley, California, the owner, Akira Akamura, told me they were using a hydrogenated oil. When I explained to Mr. Akamura that hydrogenated oils contain an ingredient now known to cause heart disease and type 2 diabetes, he changed to peanut oil for tempura and stir-fries and to extra-virgin olive oil for the delicate Japanese salads on his menu.

Mr. Akamura cares about quality and the well-being of his staff and patrons. So do restaurant owners in your neighborhood. Share what you have learned here.

Mexican restaurants usually use less partially hydrogenated oils, but they may be lurking if the restaurant is part of a chain and does not prepare its own beans, burrito fillings, meat, and chips. Many restaurant chains count on the preservative qualities of partially hydrogenated oils since their foods are often shipped from a central location a great distance away.

Again, the best thing you can do is *ask*.

Upscale and Health-Conscious Restaurants

Almost always, the better restaurants do not use partially hydrogenated vegetable oils. These are usually places where the chef is dedicated to providing delicious foods of the highest quality. The raw materials come from local gardens, free-range poultry farms, grass-fed-beef ranches, and nearby oceans, lakes, and streams. At these restaurants, the chefs are well aware of the dangers of hydrogenated oil. They also recognize the difference in taste. They wouldn't dream of using it. This can also be true in simpler local restaurants as well, where the management prides itself in serving its community with the freshest and best foods.

That is true in my small town, where there are two small restaurants. One is an all-day cafe; the other is a dinner-only restaurant. Both have knowledgeable owners and an unusually demanding clientele that knows the downside of hydrogenated vegetable oils. Both restaurants have banished partially hydrogenated vegetable oils and margarine from their kitchens.

You can accomplish this where you live, by asking questions, thus making your favorite restaurants and cafés places where you feel the safety of being well fed.

Chapter Fourteen

Inspiring Changes
at Home

It's usually difficult to begin a project that will alter a habit, especially a lifelong habit. This can be especially true of changing eating habits.

Foods have certain comfort values. Foods can soothe or trigger memories of special family occasions. Every culture has its own beloved dishes, good for stomach and soul. Fortunately, almost any traditional favorites can be found or prepared without the killer ingredient we want to avoid. But making the transition to even slightly different flavors can meet with surprising resistance.

Your family, or you yourself, for that matter, may be reluctant to move quickly. So move slowly. But don't toss this project aside or relegate it to the "maybe someday" list.

Everyone needs time to adjust to change, your family perhaps more than you. Remember, you are coming to them with the idea; they may need time to juggle the pros and cons, too. Your confidence in this plan, not your urgency, is what will ultimately communicate the common sense of it.

Children and the Others You Live With

I think it's crucial to explain to the youngsters as well as the adults your reasons for changing the dietary rules in your home. Doing so is a way to reflect your respect for and inclusion of them in an important aspect of family life.

No matter how compelling you make the idea, however, children will generally resist a change that alters routines and food preferences built up over the years. This is true of adults, too, but children are likely to be less sympathetic toward your plans for a TFA-free household. Conversely, children are not as averse to change as most parents think.

Children are not by nature impossible, cranky, or tough. If your child is a picky eater or a sullen table companion, he was allowed to become the arbiter of the dinner table, the umpire of what goes and what doesn't. As children get older, their food positions become more entrenched. It may seem impossible to change an eight-year-old's diet after he's had his way since he was two. Actually, it's not.

It is imperative for parents to prevail in food tussles— without scars. You must not get angry and you must have previously made the decision that you will not force food. How much a healthy child eats is always ultimately his or her decision.

Don't make an issue of eating; it will just give your child power in an arena where you will be the loser. If your child doesn't want to eat what is put in front of him, offer the household alternative (cereal, peanut butter sandwich, carrots, something of nutritional value of your choice). If that doesn't appeal, that should be all right with you, too. Let the child know that the household alternative is always available to eat later on if he is hungry. These are reasonable positions, and if you offer them without anger or visible frustration, you will feel confidence in your plan. After all, I'm not talking about drastic changes at the dinner table. You won't be substituting clams for hamburger or disappointing your family with soft-boiled eggs instead of the Sunday morning pancake breakfast they're used to. We're speaking of simple substitutions that will take place over the ensuing weeks and months as you choose new supermarket foods: a new cracker, a new peanut butter, a new snack food, a new frozen pizza, a chicken from your kitchen or a barbecued one from a take-out shop that cooks without hydrogenated oils, instead of one from KFC.

Skipping Meals

Children who are well-adjusted eaters are either hungry or not, and they benefit from knowing either is all right with their parents. Eating problems usually result from parents' fears about their child eating too much or too little and from a lack of understanding that it's a child's right to respond to her own signals for hunger. Pediatric experts say that it is not important that a child eat every meal or eat even every day. The trouble begins when the parent cooks a substitute for the rejected meal: a frankfurter for fish, hamburger for a lamb chop, a slice of pizza instead of the chicken everyone else is having.

It's not necessary to worry about children passing up a meal because they don't like the taste, the color, because it's different from what they have come to expect, or because they are just not hungry. For instance, when you are feeding your newborn, if your infant is well and thriving, you never worry if a feeding is skipped. Children, even infants, know their food needs and capacity.

Passing up food or skipping a meal needn't mean the child is excused from the table. Part of the family meal, whether it's a quick breakfast, a picnic lunch, or dinner, is the socialization of our children. Here we teach them the niceties of the table, even how to eat certain foods; we initiate conversation, ask them about their day at school, or follow their conversational leads. This is nutrition of the highest order, as important as that in their baked potato.

Getting Everyone on Board

Everyone responds to calm, reason, respect, and empathy. Changing the foods you eat is an important project, and everyone should be in on it. Young children, teenagers, and adults all want to discuss options. Children who feel they have a respected position within the family do not habitually sulk or disregard parental decisions, even if they initially object and argue. They can become willing participants in what will be a new family adventure. Children like to be part of a family working together for a common good. Sure, they may grouch at certain changes or impositions on their freedom, but basically they are joiners, not quitters.

You'll all have to confront some differences in taste and appearance in the nonhydrogenated foods that replace your old favorites. Expect some disappointment as you discover that there are no TFA-free Ritz crackers. There is already an almost perfect substitute: Rich crackers by a company called Hain.

With a keen eye, you and your children can find goodies and practical foods for the entire family. Your children can still have tradables in their lunch boxes (even though you might not like what they get in exchange), and bring their friends home to foods other than carrots and celery. The adult you live with can still have snacks at cocktail time. Guests don't even have to know that you've switched. The differences in your dinners, lunches, breakfasts, and picnics won't even show.

Chapter Fifteen

Living Healthier in the Twenty-First Century

It is becoming increasingly clear to the professionals who investigate food and health and nutritional theories that the best eating plan is a well-balanced diet that contains a little of everything minus TFAs.

By the nineties, we began to hear dissent about the significance of low *total* cholesterol levels and a diet low in saturated fats. Today, eminent scientists, researchers, and practicing physicians (though not all) endorse a diet that includes olive oil, eggs, and red meat two or three times a week. While that is not a complete turnaround, it represents a distinct change from the very rigid low-fat stand that was once dominant.

I believed the good-for-you margarine story in the 1950s and 1960s; everyone I know did—not only doctors, but engineers, scientists, bankers, carpenters, musicians, and philosophers as well. I fell for the chicken breast, no-more-red-meat story, so much so that one of our children had never eaten steak or beef stew at home until he was eight. I would joke with my dear friend, Judy, "What's for chicken?" I tortured my children with lentil loaves and black-bean stews more than once a week in the 1970s, recipes I was never very good at preparing and had little enthusiasm for. We had so many vegetables in the house that I had to stuff some onto my pantry shelves. Butter and egg yolks were our family poison.

There are physicians who maintain that the ideal diet is very low in fat—less than 15 percent—and high in whole grains and complex carbohydrates. This theory, while having many advocates, is losing ground daily as researchers and physicians worldwide come to understand the value of a diet that includes adequate amounts of various fats, beef and eggs included.

I know how difficult it can be in our rushed lives to add another category of concern. But you are after all considering freeing your household of TFAs and doing the best you can to let your local markets and restaurants know of the problem. Putting your good sense to work simply at home is the next step. The following guidelines should make your job a lot easier.

Good-Eating Guidelines

- Today's healthy diet recommendations support eating both moderate portions of chicken and red meat.
- Eat green, yellow, orange, and red things that grow in gardens.
- Eat moderate amounts of tiny things that you can measure by the quarter-cupful, like nuts; also seeds, beans and brown grains, like rice, barley, and oats.
- Add fish to these food choices a few times a week, and you will get essential omega-3.
- Buy beef and chicken and eggs produced without antibiotics or hormones if you can find them.
- Look for grass-fed beef. As we noted earlier, grass-fed beef has omega-3 fatty acids and doesn't suffer with the overload of omega-6 from stockyard corn feed. This means you won't have an omega-6 overload, either. As

Michael Pollan pointed out in his *New York Times Magazine* feature story, "Power Steer" (March 31, 2002), the corn diet of our cattle can "so disturb the cow's digestive process—its rumen, in particular—that it can kill the animal if not managed carefully and accompanied by antibiotics." "Corn," says Pollan, "is a mainstay of livestock diets because there is no other feed quite as cheap or plentiful: thanks to federal subsidies and ever-growing surpluses, the price of corn (in March of 2002) is 50 cents less than the cost of growing it." Pollan also cites a study in *The European Journal of Clinical Nutrition* documenting that the meat of grass-fed cattle "not only had substantially less fat . . . but that the type of fats . . . were much healthier." Pollan continues, "the unnaturally rich diet of corn is fattening [the] flesh [of the steer] in a way that . . . may compromise the health of humans who will eat him." Grass-fed beef can be somewhat difficult to find and is more expensive, but it is becoming more popular as folks begin to learn about the downsides of corn-fed cattle and the slaughtering conditions that led to our recent (December 2003) episode of bovine spongiform encephalopathy, or mad cow disease. If grass-fed beef is not available now where you live, it is possible to mail order it (see www.grassfed beef.com, or www.morrisgrassfed.com, or marinsun farms@onemain.com). There is even grass-fed lamb available from a ranch on Martha's Vineyard (Allen Sheep Farm). Supermarkets cannot always carry grass-fed beef or lamb; the quantity available is still relatively small, and supermarkets need huge availability to meet customer needs.

- Check the milk you buy. Look for a note on the container that says "No rBST." That tells you the milk is hormone-free; rBST, which stands for recombinant bovine somatotropin, is a hormone fed to cows to increase their milk production. While the FDA claims that rBST is not harmful to humans, many of us remain concerned about potential health risks.

- Check the labels of the juices you think you are purchasing as "health" drinks for yourself and your children.

As you learned earlier, most bottled and canned drinks claiming to be "juice" or "tea" drinks have sugar or high-fructose corn sweeteners added, plus water. Drinking "juice" drinks—such as Snapple 100% Juiced!,* which is mainly concentrates of apple, pear, and grape sugars plus water and has more grams of sugar than a 12-ounce can of Coca-Cola—as substitutes for milk deprives children of the calcium they need for appropriate bone development.

- If you are not already eating whole grains, add brown rice, bulgur wheat, oats, whole barley, and bread made from 100 percent whole-wheat flour, to the rotation of pastas and grains you usually use. Eat garbanzos, black beans, and lentils. These carbohydrates take longer to digest, so you'll be more satisfied and won't get as hungry as quickly as you do when you eat foods made from white flour.

Brown grains, lentils, and beans can be cooked simply with water or broth (see chart opposite for cooking times). Refrigerated, these foods will keep for a week. They can be reheated quickly to accompany chicken and salad and can be added to soup or even to an omelet.

---

* Marian Burros, *The New York Times*, September 17, 2003. "The Snapple Deal: How Sweet It Is."

COOKING TIMES FOR GRAINS

Grain (per cup)	Cooking Liquid	Cooking Time	Yield
Bulgur wheat	2 cups	15 to 25 minutes	2½ cups
Couscous	1½ cups	10 minutes	3 cups
Cracked wheat	2¼ cups	2 hours	2¾ cups
Hulled barley	4 cups	2 hours	3½ cups
Pearl barley	3¼ cups	45 minutes–1 hour	3½ cups
Wheat berries	2½ cups	2½ hours	2¾ cups

Note: Soaking hulled barley, cracked wheat, or wheat berries for 5 hours or overnight will reduce cooking time. To cook bulgur wheat or couscous, pour boiling liquid over the grain, cover, and steep. Fluff with a fork.

Grain (per cup)	Cooking Liquid	Cooking Time	Yield
Buckwheat groats	2 cups	15 to 20 minutes	2½ cups
Buckwheat kasha	2 cups	10 to 12 minutes	2½ cups
Cornmeal	4 cups	10 to 15 minutes	3 to 4 cups
Millet	3 cups	30 to 40 minutes	3½ cups
Quinoa	2 cups	15 to 20 minutes	4 cups
Rice (white)	2 cups	30 minutes	2½ cups
Rice (brown)	2¼ cups	1 hour	2½ cups
Rye flakes	3 cups	1 hour	3 cups
Wild rice	2½ to 3 cups	1¼ hours	2¾ cups

- If you are watching your calories, you already know to snack on vegetables and fruit, and cut down on bread, potatoes, rice, and cake and other rich desserts. But you don't have to give up rich treats entirely. Order a hot-fudge sundae or piece of cheesecake if you must, then share it. (We almost always order a dessert when out with friends or our children but usually just one or two for the table—and several spoons.) Invent desserts with more fruit. Share a steak with a friend. Buy ten ounces of

salmon and serve it to two. Eat doubles of salad and vegetables. Be inventive with snacks (see page 89). And never forsake your favorite martini, glass of wine, or celebratory champagne.
- Always exercise.

Cooking Suggestions for Grains

Grains can be delicious and interesting. To add variety to the grains you cook, consider the following suggestions.

- Use vegetable or chicken stock as the cooking liquid, or add 1 to 2 teaspoons of soy sauce or Asian sesame oil and some chopped onion to the cooking liquid.
- Sauté finely chopped onion, shallots, or garlic and add before cooking the grain.
- Experiment with spices, for instance, add ground cinnamon to rice and chili flakes to millet.
- Crumble in dried herbs before cooking.
- Add minced fresh herbs after cooking.
- Add chopped dried fruit, such as apricot, or finely chopped celery sautéed in liquid to rice.
- For a meatless meal, fold freshly toasted walnuts and sautéed mushrooms into cooked barley, rice, or wheat berries. Wheat berries are a nice substitute for the chewiness of meat.
- Add leftover slivered chicken, green peas, and olive oil flavored with herbs to rice.
- Add herbs, such as parsley or cilantro, to chopped scallions, chopped red onion, or chopped spinach or chard. These colorful additions can be prepared while the grain is cooking.
- Sprinkle on olive oil.

The Importance of Weight and Exercise in a Healthy Diet

While this is not a book about managing your weight, weight is a crucial national problem and has become an epidemic that I think deserves mention in any book about food, especially a book about fats and health. Despite what seems like the country's obsession with professional sports; with hiking, biking, and skiing; with a multibillion-dollar weight-control industry; with glossy magazines that portray fourteen-year-old, eighty-five-pound models as the ideal physical type; America has gone fat.

Earlier in the book we discussed the link between diets high in TFAs, obesity, heart disease, and type 2 diabetes. If you consume too many calories you'll become fat. If you don't exercise, you will become fatter still. A November 11, 2003, article in *The New York Times* states, "In 2000, for the first time, the number of overweight people in the world rose to match the number who were underweight and starving." According to a 2003 announcement by the Centers for Disease Control, "Obesity may be overtaking smoking as a cause of death in the United States." James Hill, the dean of American obesity studies at the University of Colorado, says that "if obesity is left unchecked almost all Americans will be overweight within a few generations."

It's not just us. Supersize junk food is replacing traditional diets everywhere. For instance, *USA Today* on November 18, 2003, reported that throughout Europe, more than half of adults are overweight and up to 30 percent are obese; in Italy, 36 percent of children ages six through ten are overweight. That, says Greg Critser in his March 2000 *Harper's magazine* article, is a "key reason why Eli Lilly and Company, the seventy-five billion dollar pharmaceutical company, is building the largest factory in history dedicated to the production of a single drug."

That drug is insulin, the pharmaceutical answer to what happens when exercise is absent and the sugars, high fats, and white flour of our national diet have destroyed the pancreas's insulin-producing ability. The relationship between poor diet and type 2 diabetes is so clear, so strong, that a new term has even been coined in the medical literature: *diabesity*. Our children are growing up on this processed-food diet, and many of them will need to take pills to manage their diabetes. James Kappel of Eli Lilly said, somewhat nonchalantly, in his interview with Greg Critser, "You've just got to be in diabetes."

It is particularly stunning that, despite the significant shifts in our understanding of the basics of a healthy lifestyle in the last ten years, especially of the importance of exercise and the benefits of monounsaturated oil, the USDA Food Pyramid—the one hanging in most every school and clinic in the country—has not been revised in over a decade. Looking to update public awareness, the nonprofit nutrition science organization, Oldways Preservation Trust, in consultation with Walter Willett, M.D., and the staff at the Harvard School of Public Health, developed its own food pyramid, which it calls the EatWise Pyramid (see figure 1 on page 117).

Take a look at the two pyramids and you will see notable differences. Look first at the wide bottom layer of the EatWise Pyramid, the layer representing the most important element of our diets. In contrast to the USDA pyramid (figure 2 on page 118), which advocates eating a diet consisting primarily of simple carbohydrate foods like white rice, bread, and pasta, at the wide bottom layer the EatWise Pyramid advocates a bottom line of exercise. Yes, exercise in a food pyramid! As a basis for healthy bodies, daily exercise, Walter Willett maintains, is as essential as healthy foods. For carbohydrates, the

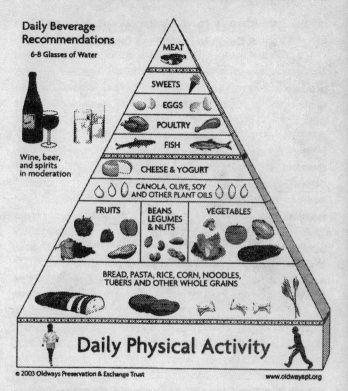

Daily Beverage Recommendations

6-8 Glasses of Water

Wine, beer, and spirits in moderation

MEAT

SWEETS

EGGS

POULTRY

FISH

CHEESE & YOGURT

CANOLA, OLIVE, SOY AND OTHER PLANT OILS

FRUITS | BEANS LEGUMES & NUTS | VEGETABLES

BREAD, PASTA, RICE, CORN, NOODLES, TUBERS AND OTHER WHOLE GRAINS

Daily Physical Activity

© 2003 Oldways Preservation & Exchange Trust

www.oldwayspt.org

Fig. 1. Eatwise Pyramid

EatWise Pyramid suggests eating a variety of *whole* grains. Its middle section offers a hierarchy of fruits and vegetables, oils, dairy products, fish, poultry, eggs, and sweets. Notably, plant oils are not lumped together with other fats and oils at the top of the pyramid but rather reside in the middle because, as we now know, they are important to our health. I think you'll find that the EatWise Pyramid offers much clearer and more up-to-date guidelines for maintaining optimal health. You might

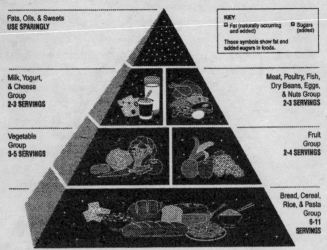

Fig. 2. USDA Food Guide Pyramid

want to download a beautiful color version from the Oldways website (www.oldwayspt.org) and keep it handy.

Exercise is the crucial link for improved well-being. It is even more critical for the physical, intellectual, and emotional development of children, who need adult guidance in this arena just as they need guidance in what they eat, smoke, and drink, who their friends are, and how they study. Currently, however, only one state, Illinois, requires physical education for all grades, kindergarten through twelfth.

Exercise is forsaken when we hurtle from house to car to activity to car to shop to car to eat to car and home. It's much harder to incorporate walking into a day that is programmed with pickups and deliveries and more time at the computer. It's much harder to incorporate physical activity in days that are rushed with deadlines for everything.

Technology is sexier than exercise. So activities like computer games or television watching—with its child-focused junk-food advertising—take its place, captivating, stunning, and blunting children's imaginations. Television advertising to adults consoles with pills that can cure multiple ills, encouraging complacency and the false security that the pills will make up for our sedentary lifestyles. And while we enjoy our sedentary lifestyles, we nibble and nosh from an endless stream of cellophane bags and fast-food meals. We don't even have to get up to change the channel or answer our phones.

That's why planned exercise times are more important now than ever.

Creative Exercise

If you don't have time for some form of regular exercise, are not a person who can walk to work or to shopping near home or meet your children on foot after school, look for other ways you can fit in even a little exercise. Press to make room for the following moments of activity in your schedule:

- Use the stairs in your office or apartment building rather than the elevator.
- Look for stairs everywhere. Use them.
- Walk a bit after dinner; even fifteen minutes will benefit you, your children, and friends. Do your best to walk to accomplish chores. If you can, choose a neighborhood cleaner and shoe repair shop rather than ones on the other side of town that you'd have to drive to.
- Select restaurants you can walk to and from.

- Park some distance from wherever you are going.
- Leave the subway or bus a stop or two early, or park your car a block or two from work.
- Keep a Frisbee or a soccer ball and your sneakers in the car. With the equipment available, you will see more opportunities for activity.
- If you shop at a mall, make the time for a lap or two after you finish your shopping. If you walk moderately fast, you may get a mile in before you leave.

A Cautionary Tale

On an island named Kosrae, the smallest of four island states that make up the federated states of Micronesia, a new epidemic that some epidemiologists call the New World Syndrome is dramatically shortening life expectancy. We might expect that it would be famine or diseases like AIDS or malaria that are reducing that population, but in fact it is indiscriminate Westernization and the destruction of traditional behavior (exercise and diet) and culture that is ruining the health and stability of Kosraeans.

In the June 2001 issue of the *Atlantic,* Ellen Ruppel-Shell describes the insidious transformation of this formerly self-sufficient island culture. The people on this small island used to earn their living from small-plot family farming, from the growing of bananas, papayas, multiple varieties of taro, breadfruit, coconut, and from lots of rockfish fishing. Now they drive to computer jobs mainly in cramped, hot offices and have alarmingly high rates of heart disease, type 2 diabetes, and high blood pressure. Why?

In Kosrae, everyone used to walk. Now, says Ms. Shell, "to walk is to announce that one is too poor to ride." Before these prosperous times, Kosraens ate local products; now there has been a massive invasion of prepared and processed hydrogenated vegetable oil-containing food from the United States, Australia, and New Zealand. As in so many other places around the globe, the ability to purchase imported packaged foods demonstrates that you have money. It is more prestigious to serve Oreo cookies than fresh coconut. The variety of food laden with hydrogenated vegetable oil goes like this: frozen turkey tails ready for a Crisco frying, Lay's potato chips, ramen noodles, Ritz crackers, Spam, Oreos, cakes, and candies. Margarine and Crisco are used in bread products, and donuts, which are fried in hydrogenated canola or corn oil.

Not only are the Kosraeans sick, they are also obese. The same thing that causes their obesity—a diet high in poor-quality foods and the loss of lifestyle-driven physical activity—leads to most of the illness the overwhelmed island doctors now have to cope with.

Another South Pacific Island, Nauru, a former farm culture, under whose farms phosphate was discovered and depleted by foreign mining companies, is now also a Westernized office culture. Are they enjoying prosperity? Yes. Some Western luxuries? Yes. But as Stephen Auerback, M.D., a New York epidemiologist says, along with their wealth, "the worst of manufactured American food culture has landed. Gobs of hydrogenated fat, sugar, refined starches . . . the worst of 1950s cuisine"—and the highest obesity rates and diabetes rates in the world.

Chapter Sixteen

Does Action Work Faster Than Education?

A Modest Proposal

Education happens slowly, especially if the object of the education will have a major economic impact on powerful industry. Action eliminates the problem sooner. You and the vast community of people who are rapidly coming to know the dangers of TFAs have the power to influence industry by boycotting all products with partially hydrogenated oils. Your boycott can be powerful—and successful.

A triumphant boycott is thrilling. A triumphant boycott squashes the special interest groups that influence and manipulate the congressional vote. Remember the California grape picker's success? When people in California stopped buying grapes from farms and vineyards that did not pay union wages, the grape industry was nearly decimated until it relented.

Nothing is more successful in the domain of business than consumers demonstrating their power by where, and on what, they spend their dollars. Business needs your continued patronage. You are the determining factor, the link between product production and financial success. It is imperative for industry to catch up to your demands, to follow your lead.

It can be daunting to consider taking on megabusiness, but

your power as a consumer really *can* change the way corporate giants behave. Their bottom line is to make the profit as large as possible by making their product as appealing as possible (price, packaging, taste). If you stop purchasing Wheat Thins or fried fast foods and don't even begin to purchase new TFA-loaded products that keep coming to the market, such as Quaker Chewy Granola Bars or Skippy Squeeze Stix, industry will notice and will want to know why. Choosing *not* to buy such products will force manufacturers to change the fat in their recipes, and the fast-food industry to reconsider the use of hydrogenated oils in theirs.

We all wish for guardians to safeguard our health. Unfortunately, we must take on certain health concerns ourselves. Can you imagine thousands and thousands and thousands of shoppers leaving hydrogenated packages behind? And thousands of shoppers becoming millions? Shunning muffins, and donuts, and fast-food culprits, and cookies, and cakes, and crackers with hydrogenated oils? Our determination and indignation will drive this campaign. And if we turn out forcefully, our health concerns might even become the concerns of Congress.

And it has to be we who move. Most politicians don't care enough, and those few who do can rarely muster the votes to effect change. As an example, in July 2002, the week that the Institute of Medicine finally reported the result of their investigations (that no level of TFA is safe), a bill by California representative Deborah Bowen, requiring listing the presence of dangerous TFAs on food labels in California, was defeated in committee. In an e-mail to colleagues that afternoon, Jeffrey Aron, M.D., a professor of medicine at the University of California, San Francisco, who has been fighting the presence of TFAs for years, wrote that he "hoped that this irony was not lost on our trusted representatives." Health issues left to congressional maneuvering frequently end up like this. Now, of course, since the Institute of Medicine's report has initiated the long-awaited mandate from the FDA regarding nationwide labeling by January, 2006, California will not have to take care of itself.

How Will Our Markets Look When We Succeed?

Our markets will look the same. The packaging will undoubtedly be as colorful. It will be easy to see what's good for us to eat and what's not because there will be a label across the front of the package—not a warning label, but an informational label that reads: "This product does not contain partially hydrogenated vegetable oil." Our success would allow us more comfort about what we buy and feed our families, and about what our families are eating when they're not at home. New recipes would be developed using fats and oils friendly to our bodies. Even with moderate success, many manufacturers would revise their recipes and partially hydrogenated vegetable oil would be replaced with pure, unrefined vegetable oils or with butter, as several food manufacturers in the vanguard of change have already done. Among these are Adrienne's Gourmet Foods, Almondina, Amy's, Barbara's Bakery, Hain, Newman's Own Organics, and the other producers whose names are listed in Appendix B.

While some businesses would continue to use partially hydrogenated vegetable oils for years to come, we will be alert and their products will stand out on the market shelves, naked without their identifying label: "This product does not contain partially hydrogenated vegetable oil."

In a perfect, moral, and responsible world, Congress would take on the role of public health guardian. In a perfect world, our Surgeon General would recognize the dangers of TFAs and their relationship to the epidemic of obesity. In our less-than-perfect world, Congress has not voted to ban advertisements of food with partially hydrogenated vegetable oils; nor, are they working toward a ban of junk-food advertising on television aimed at children—even though it is our government that declared TFAs a danger and ordered the packaging mandate. In a *really* perfect world, Congress would ban partially hydrogenated vegetable oils from food. In this real world, we have work to accomplish.

Become Active in Your Children's School

What do your children eat at school? If left to Francine Kaufman, M.D., all schools would have instructions for children (and their parents) about healthy eating, and no school would be allowed to accept fast food and sweetened drinks as lunch or recess options, or to display advertising for those products. (Telephone conversation, February 21, 2001.)

Some experts blame obesity and the subsequent childhood type 2 diabetes epidemic on schools for cutting physical education programs and stocking school cafeterias and vending machines with junk food, fast food, and sugar drinks, and for installing Channel One, a free "educational" TV service available in schools that accepts commercial advertising for colas and sugared cereals with TFAs, to name just two foods. In the January 5, 2004 issue of *Pediatrics,* a position paper from the American Academy of Pediatrics states that soft drinks should be eliminated from schools to help handle the nation's obesity epidemic and that "physicians should contact superintendents and school board members and emphasize . . . that every school . . . shares a responsibility for the nutritional health of its students." California has already taken a giant step and is a leader in eliminating unhealthy drinks in public schools. Beginning in July of 2004 no elementary school or middle school will be able to sell sugared drinks during school hours."*

Perhaps the soccer uniforms and fancy scoreboards paid for by Coca-Cola and Taco Bell will have to go, especially if the California mandate is extended to high school. These solutions, to stop fast-food and sugared drinks in schools, do present the next problem, as all solutions to problems do—will the loss of junk food and soft drink funding stifle athletic programs as state budgets for schools continue to slide? Will extracurricular activities disappear from the calendar? Can we count on parents to take up enough of the slack so that the loss of luxuries the industry provides doesn't cause programs and school teams to evaporate?

Here is a thought for influencing industry in another way. McDonald's, Burger King, Taco Bell, KFC, Coca-Cola, Snapple, and Pepsi do not want to give up their position to capture our children as consumers. Let's give them an opportunity to stay, but *only* with foods and drinks that support healthy eating. Why not petition fast-food companies and drink manufacturers to invest in the development of foods and drinks that meet the criteria of health professionals and concerned parents? That way there could be a win for everyone. Junk food in schools would transform into healthy food, and industry, delighted to obtain school contracts, would continue to support football uniforms and music teachers. How wonderful if Taco Bell invented a new green salad with sliced and poached—not fried—chicken decorated with TFA-free whole wheat croutons and shavings of TFA-free cheese. And there is a drink in the marketplace that fizzes and has no added sugar; it's called Fizzy Lizzy and comes in many flavors. Is that sort of in-

---

* "New Warnings on Soda," *Chronicle*, January 9, 2004, Editorial Page A22.

vention beyond Coca-Cola? Given the nature of the world in general, we all are pressed to become advocates of one thing or another. At least *we* can aim for what we want, and perhaps you can influence your children's school to rethink its position, as well.

Become Active in Your Community

On a large sign above the food counters, the University Hospital cafeteria in New York City declares that its food is trans fat free. What is your local hospital feeding its patients and its staff? What are the visitors eating?

Legal Sea Foods, a restaurant that originated in Boston and now has several restaurants around the country, announces on its menu that all its food is trans fat free. The CEO of Legal Seafoods, Roger Berkowitz, is a member of the Harvard School of Public Health's Nutrition Roundtable. Mr. Berkowitz first addressed his fish-frying oils, moved to perfecting a frying oil for potatoes, and then found a new supplier for the restaurant's oyster crackers. Restaurants can do this.

Does your local Lamaze group suggest the elimination of hydrogenated oils? What's for lunch at senior centers where you live? What's served at college cafeterias where your children go to school and where perhaps you teach? What are the babies being fed at day care centers, and young children at preschools? Have you noticed what's in the public schools' prepared food?

Take a Stand at Fast-Food Places

You already know that most food items in most fast-food places are made with hydrogenated oils. Go in anyway and ask about them. Then register your disappointment, and let them know you are leaving without buying lunch. This kind

of protest makes a huge impression on processed-food manufacturers and on fast-food giants like Burger King, KFC, and
Taco Bell.

McDonald's and other big fast-food names have in the past
bent to demands from consumers. Sometimes the changes
support good eating, sometimes not. When there was a
protest in the 1980s against using tropical oils and beef tallow
to fry potatoes (at the time, consumer advocates erroneously
thought that tropical oils and beef tallow were bad for your
health), McDonald's moved to using domestic oils to satisfy
their customers. Unfortunately, the move was to hydrogenated domestic oils (corn, safflower, soybean, canola, sunflower) and the American diet was the worse for it, this time
as a result of consumer-advocate support. A pertinent discus-
sion in an article in *The Lancet*, March 6, 1993, shows that as
the U.S. fast-food industry discarded beef tallow from their
french fry recipe in the early 1990s and moved to partially hydrogenated vegetable oils, the percentage of trans fatty acids
increased from 3–5 percent to about 30 percent.

Make your voice heard, and discover the community of
folks who care as much as you do about the health of the nation. You help create the legacy we hand down. Make yours
one you can be proud of.

APPENDIX A

WORST OFFENDER FOODS

Following is a list of the most common hideouts for TFAs. The list is general and contains products you'll find prepackaged in markets and freshly prepared in bakeries, restaurants, and wherever food is sold. Remember, *always read labels* and be on the lookout for margarine as an ingredient. Margarine, which is often laden with TFAs, is frequently used in packaged foods.

BAKED GOODS

Biscuit, cake, muffin, and pie crust mixes
Bread
Cakes (assorted types, including frosted and
    decorated birthday cakes)
Cookies
Donuts
Frosting mixes and canned frostings
Muffins
Pastries
Pie crusts
Pies
Pizza crusts (ready to bake)

FAST FOOD

Breakfast cakes (such as cinnamon buns and Danish pastry)
Croutons (and other salad crispies)
Desserts (brownies, cookies, cakes, pies)
Donuts
Flour tortillas
French fries (and other fried and grilled potatoes)
Fried onion rings
Fried tortillas
Hamburger and hot dog buns
Nuggets (such as breaded chicken nuggets and breaded potato nuggets)
Sauces
Soups

FROZEN FOODS

Breaded foods (such as fish sticks and potato nuggets)
Burritos
French fries (and other fried and grilled potatoes)
Frozen dinners and side dishes
Pizza
Pot pies
Pot stickers
Quiches

PACKAGED MEALS AND MEAL HELPERS

Dessert toppings
    Flavored sauces
    Whipped
Egg substitutes

Gravy mixes
Packaged stove-top meal helpers
Quick-cooking rice, potato, and pasta side dishes
Soups (including reduced-fat soups)
   Canned soups
   Instant dry soup mixes
   Instant soup in a cup
   Ramen (TFAs are in the spice mix)

PANTRY STAPLES

Baby foods (such as teething crackers)
Bread
Butterlike spreads
Canned and dry soups
Cereals
Chips
Cookie mixes and prepared cookie dough
Cookies
Crackers
Croutons
Frosting mixes
Margarine
Nondairy creamers
Peanut butter
Vegetable oil shortenings

SNACK FOODS

Bar snacks (such as pretzel-nut mixes, fried sesame sticks, fried green peas)
Breath mints
Candies (boxed, wrapped, and sold in bulk)
Cereal ("health") bars

Chips
Cookies
Crackers
Dips for chips
Donuts
Microwave popcorn
Nuts that are roasted or fried
Pretzels
Snack packs (such as crackers and peanut butter)

APPENDIX B

TRANS FAT–FREE FOOD LIST

Following is a list of some of the packaged foods I have found that are TFA-free. Use the list as a guide, always seeking new additions and checking ingredient lists. Sometimes manufacturers of a TFA-free food will make other varieties that contain partially hydrogenated vegetable oil—including some of those manufacturers listed here—so it's imperative that you develop the habit of reading labels.

Many snack foods, bakery items, health bars, and even some cereals with carefully crafted names that imply they are good for you ("natural" or "healthy") are places where partially hydrogenated vegetable oils commonly lurk. Be particularly careful when shopping for these foods. And take note: Products that are free of trans fats may still be high in various sugars. There may also be other ingredients you'd like to eliminate from your diet, such as MSG, fractionated palm oil, and hydrolized protein. So shop wisely, and remember: The ingredients list is the place to look.

There is no shortage of packaged foods that are delicious and consistent with healthy eating. By shopping selectively you can enjoy flavor and variety without sacrificing your good health.

BREADS AND BAKED GOODS

Alvarado Street Bakery
Bagels
Sprouted Sourdough bread
Sprouted Wheat Burger buns
Sprouted Wheat Raisin bread
100% Whole Wheat Oatmeal bread

Bakers Delight
Crumpets

Beckman's
French Whole Wheat bread
German Farm bread
Oat Bran bread
Pure Rye bread
Sourdough bread
Swiss 3-Seed bread

Brother Juniper's
Cinnamon-Raisin bread
Multi-Grain Whole Wheat bread
Roasted 3-Seed sandwich buns
Struan bread
Wild Rice and Onion sandwich
  buns

Campbell Bread Baking Company
Carrot Raisin bread
French Butter croissant
Oatbran bread
Peasant White bread
Pumpkin bread
Split-Top Buttermilk bread
Whole Wheat croissant
Zucchini bread

Colombo
Extra Sour French bread

Earth Grains
Buttermilk bread
Potato bread
Whole Wheat bread

Francisco
Round Sourdough bread

Hazelsauer
Mixed Grain bread
Sunflower Organic German bread
Two-Grain bread
Whole Rye bread
Whole-Grain Organic
  German bread

Home Pride
Wheat bread

Iron Kids
No Crust bread
Round Top bread
Wheat bread

Lender's
Plain bagels

Mi Rancho
Corn tortillas

Oroweat bagels
Country Potato
Health Nut
Plain

Oroweat breads
Honey Wheat Berry
Oatnut 3-Seed
Russian Rye

Otis Spunkmeyer muffins
Almond Poppy Seed
Banana Nut
Chocolate Chocolate Chip

Rudi's Organic Bakery
Cinnamon Raisin bread
Colorado Cracked Wheat bread
Multi-Grain Oat bread
Rocky Mountain Sourdough bread

Sara Lee
Homestyle Wheat bread
Honey White bread

Sconehenge
English muffins
Scones (assorted flavors)

Stone Mill Farms
European Style Wheat bread
Honey Wheat Berry
Stoneground 100% Whole Wheat
   bread

Tea-n-Crumpets
Organic crumpets

Thomas' English Muffins
Honey Wheat
Original
Sourdough

Thomas' New York Style Bagels
Cinnamon Raisin Swirl
Plain

Thomas' Sahara pita bread
White
Whole Wheat

Vital Vittles
Cinnamon Honey buns
Cornbread
Flax Seed Oat bread
Raisin bread
3-Seed bread

Wonder Bread
White

BUTTER AND BUTTERLIKE SPREADS

*Earth Balance Natural Buttery
   Sticks*

Spectrum
Natural Spread
Organic margarine

Vermont Butter & Cheese Company
Cultured butter

CEREALS

Arrowhead Mills
Kamut Flakes
Maple Buckwheat Flakes
Shredded Wheat
Spelt Flakes

Barbara's Bakery
Apple Cinnamon Toasted O's
Bite-Sized Shredded Oats
   (assorted flavors)
Honey Nut Toasted O's
Multigrain Shredded Spoonfuls
Puffins (assorted flavors)
Shredded Wheat

Cascadian Farm
Honey Nut O's
Multi Grain Squares
Oats & Honey Granola
Purely O's

EnviroKidz
Organic Cheetah Chomps
Organic Gorilla Munch
Organic Koala Crisp
Organic Peanut Butter
   Panda Puffs

General Mills Cheerios
Original

General Mills Chex
Corn Chex
Rice Chex
Wheat Chex

Health Valley
Blueberry Bliss
Organic Amaranth Flakes
Organic Golden Flax
Organic Oat Bran Flakes
Rice Crunch-Ems!

Kashi
Good Friends Cinna-Raisin Crunch
Heart to Heart
Organic Promise Autumn Wheat
Organic Promise
   Cranberry Sunshine
Puffed Kashi

Kellogg's
Raisin Bran
Rice Krispies
Special K

Nature's Path
Flax Plus
Ginger Zing Granola
Heritage Bites
Heritage O's
Millet Rice Oatbran Flakes
Muesli
Organic Hemp Plus Granola

Peace Cereal
Cinnamon Apple Crisp
Mango Passion Crisp
Raspberry Ginger Crisp
Vanilla Almond Crisp

Post
Bran Flakes
Grape Nuts
Shredded Wheat

Quaker
Oat Bran
Puffed Rice
Puffed Wheat

Uncle Sam Cereal
Wheat Flakes
Whole Wheat with Flax Seed

Weetabix
Organic Whole Grain Wheat Cereal

CHIPS, PRETZELS, AND OTHER SNACKS

Barbara's Bakery
Cheese puff bakes (assorted flavors)
Cheese puffs (assorted flavors)
Potato chips (assorted flavors)

Bearitos Tortilla Chips
Blue Tortilla Chips
Unsalted Yellow Corn
Yellow Corn

Boulder Potato Company Chips
Jalapeño Cheddar
Malt Vinegar and Sea Salt
Totally Natural

Cape Cod
Jalapeño and Aged Cheddar
  potato chips
Sea Salt and Vinegar
  potato chips

Corn Cheaps
Organic White Corn
Organic Yellow Corn

Eden Vegetable Chips
Seaweed

Fall River Wild Rice Chips
Garlic
Lightly Salted

Frito Lay Potato Chips
Lay's Classic
Ruffles Original
Wavy Lay's

Garden of Eatin' Tortilla Chips
Black Bean Chili
Blue Chips No Salt Added
Chili and Lime
Red Hot Blues
Tamari
Yellow Corn

GeniSoy Soy Crisps
Deep Sea Salted
Roasted Garlic & Onion
Zesty Barbecue

Good Health Potato Chips
Black Pepper Olive Oil
Garlic in Olive Oil
Rosemary
Trio in Olive Oil

Guiltless Gourmet Tortilla Chips
Baked Chili Lime
Baked Mucho Nacho
Baked Organic Blue Corn
Baked Sweet White Corn
Baked Unsalted Yellow Corn

Hain
Carrot Chips
Mini Rice Snack Munchies (assorted
  varieties)
Soy Munchies (assorted varieties)

Lundberg Family Farms
Bean and Rice Chips (assorted
  varieties)
Brown Rice Chips (assorted varieties)
Organic Whole Grain Rice Cakes
  (assorted varieties)

Kettle Krisps Potato Chips
Lightly Salted
Mustard and Honey
New York Cheddar with Herbs
Sea Salt and Vinegar

Kettle Tortilla Chips
Blue Corn Organic
Five Grain Yellow Corn Organic

Sesame Blue Moons
Sweet Brown Rice & Black Bean
  Organic

Pringles
Original
Salt and Vinegar

M. Season's Potato Chips
Honey Barbeque (reduced fat)
Ranch Ripple (reduced fat)
Yogurt and Green Onion
  (reduced fat)

Mexi-Snax Tortilla Chips
Nacho Cheese
Pico de Gallo
Sesame
Tamari

Native Kjalii Tortilla Chips
Fresh-Cut White and Yellow
  Corn, thin
Fresh-Cut White Corn, thick

Newman's Own Organics
Pretzel Nuggets
Salted Pretzel Sticks
Spelt Pretzels
Tortilla Chips
Unsalted Rounds Pretzels

Que Pasa Tortilla Chips
Organic Blue Corn
Organic White Corn
Organic Yellow Corn

Robert's American Gourmet
Original Potato Flyers

Rold Gold Pretzels
Braided Twists
Classic Sticks
Classic Tiny Twists Pretzels

RW Garcia Tortilla Chips
Organic Black Bean Garlic
Organic Blues
Yellow Salted

Sensible Foods Cracklin' Fruit
  100% crunch-dried fruit bits
Cherry Berry
  (Apples, Blueberries, Cherries,
  Strawberries)
Orchard
  (Apples, Apricots, Peaches)
Tropical
  (Apples, Pineapples, Mangoes,
  Bananas)

Skinny Corn Chips
Barbeque
Nacho Cheese
Original
Sour Cream & Onion

Snyder's of Hanover
Mini pretzels
Olde Tyme pretzels
Organic Pumpernickel and
  Onion pretzels
Sourdough Nibblers

Sun Chips
Original

Terra
Blues
Exotic Vegetable chips

Potpourri potato chips
Red Bliss potato chips
Sweet Potato chips
Taro chips
Yukon Gold potato chips

Westbrae
Sesame Brown Rice Wafers

William Poll Baked Potato Thins
Garlic
Onion
Rosemary

Yamamoto
Seaweed Chips

COOKIES

Barbara's
Chocolate Chip Crisp
Fig Bars
Old-Fashioned Oatmeal Crisp
Traditional Shortbread Crisp

Bastoncini
Crisp Raisin Cookies

Beth's Cookies
Chocolate Chip
Oatmeal Currant
Shortenin' Bread
Triple Ginger Snaps

Bonne Maman
Butter Cookies

Country Choice
Chocolate Chip Walnut
Ginger Snaps

Oatmeal Chocolate Chip
Vanilla Sandwich Cremes
Vanilla Wafers

Cougar Mountain Gourmet Cookies
Butterscotch Oatmeal
Chewy Molasses-Ginger

Emily's Bakery
Almond Macadamia
Chocolate Chip Almond

Frankly Natural
Coconut
Peanut Butter
Vegan Apricot Almond
Vegan Double Carob
Vegan Peanut Butter

Hain
Animal Cookies (lowfat)
Animal Grahams
Chocolate Animal Grahams

Health Valley
Amaranth Graham
Apricot Bakes (fat-free)
Date Bakes (fat-free)
Oat Bran Graham
Oatmeal Peanut Crunch

Health Valley Café Creations
Chocolate Chip
Raisin Oatmeal

Heaven Scent
Almond Windmill
Apricot Fruit Flip
Spice Windmill

Immaculate Baking Company
Leapin' Lemon
Pumpkin Gingerlies
Raspberry Brambles

Lady J's Cookies
Date Pecan
Oatmeal Raisin
Peanut Butter Pecan

Lady Walton Wafers
Amaretto White Chocolate
Chocolate Raspberry
Creamy Dark Chocolate

Lotus Bakery
Ginger Snap
Oatmeal Raisin
Orange Chocolate Chip
Peanut Butter
Tahini Coconut

Mariapple Cookies
Ginger Snaps (fat-free)
Oatmeal (fat-free)
Peanut Butter (fat-free)

Mi-Del
Honey Grahams
Pecan Cookies

Monster Cookie
Chocolate Chip
Oatmeal
Peanut Butter

Mrs. Denson's
Chocolate Chip Macaroon
Oatmeal Raisin
Quinoa Macaroon

Newman's Own Organics
Alphabet Cookies
Champion Chip Cookies
Fig Newmans
Ginger-O's
Newman-O's

Pamela's Products
Almond Anise Biscotti
Chocolate Chunk Pecan
  Shortbread
Chocolate Walnut Biscotti
Oatmeal Date Coconut
Peanut Butter Cookies

St. Amour Cookies
Chocolate Peanut Butter
  (low-fat)
Cinnamon (low-fat)
Orange Chocolate Chip
  (low-fat)

Sunflour Bakery
Chocolate Chip
Peanut Butter

Trader Joe's
Chocolate Almond Biscotti

Walker's
Fine Oatcakes
Shortbread (assorted)

Westbrae Cookies
Classic Chocolate Chip
Cookie Jar Oatmeal Raisin

CRACKERS

Adrienne's Lavosh-Hawaii
Caraway Rye
Classic Island
Peppercorn

Ak-Mak Crackers

Barbara's
Cheese Bites
Original Rite Lite Rounds
Tamari Sesame Rite Lite Rounds
Wheatines

Blue Diamond Nut Thins
Almond
Hazelnut
Smokehouse

*Courtney's Fine English
   Water Crackers*
Classic Flavour
Cracked Pepper
Sun-Dried Tomato

Crostini Tuscan Crackers
Olive Oil
Rosemary
Stoneground Wheat

Devonsheer
Classic Original Water
   Crackers
Melba Rounds
Mini Sesame Water Crackers

Eden Rice Crackers
Nori Maki
Tamari

Edward and Sons Rice Snaps
Cheddar
Tamari Sesame
Toasted Onion

Finn Crisp
Rye Crispbread

Good Health
Cheddar Guppies

Guiltless Gourmet UFO's
Original
Roasted Garlic

Hain
Crispettes
Oyster
Wheatettes

Haute Cuisine Crackers
Basil Pepper
Roasted Onion
Saffron

Health Valley
Bruschetta Vegetable Crackers
Corn Bread Crackers
Cracked Pepper
Low-Fat French Onion Crackers
Sesame
Stoned Wheat

John W.M. Macy's
Melting Parmesan Cheese
   Sticks

Kashi TLC (Tasty Little Crackers)
Country Cheddar
Honey Sesame

Natural Ranch
Original 7-Grain

Kavli Crispbread
5-Grain
Hearty Thick

Partners Crackers
Fresh Garlic
Pepper Melange

Manischewitz Matzo

Real Foods
Organic Corn Thins
Organic Multi-Grain Thins

Ryvita
Fat-Free Fruit Crunch
Whole Grain Light Rye Crackers
Whole Grain Sesame Rye

Starr Ridge Crackers
Asiago Cheese
Garlic Herb
Olive Oil
Parmesan Cheese
Red Onion with Pistachio
   and Asiago Cheese
Walnut

Trader Joe's
Cocktail Crackers
Corn Tortilla Flat Bread
   (assorted varieties)

Wasa Crispbread
Fiber Rye
Light Rye
Soya

Westbrae
Ry Crisp Natural

FROZEN FOODS

Amy's
All American Burger
   (vegetarian)
Apple Pie
Black Bean Vegetable Enchilada
Broccoli Pot Pie
Chili and Cornbread
Macaroni & Cheese
Mexican Tamale Pie
Pizza (assorted varieties)
Santa Fe Enchilada Bowl
Vegetable Lasagne

Boca
Burgers (vegan)
Meatless Breakfast Links
Meatless Chik'n Patties
Meatless Italian Sausages

Cascadian Farm
Country Herb Chicken
Pasta Primavera
Spinach Lasagne

Cedarlane
Spinach and Feta Pie
Stuffed Mediterranean Foccacia

DiGiorno Pizza
Four-Cheese
Pepperoni

Donna's Tamales
Assorted varieties

Freschetta Brick Oven Pizza
Italian Style Pepperoni
Roasted Portabella Mushrooms &
 Spinach

Healthy Choice
Beef Merlot
Chicken Parmigiana
Grilled Chicken Marinara
Oriental-Style Beef

*Kellogg's Eggo Special K
 Fat-Free Waffles*

Lean Cuisine
Chicken Fettucini with Broccoli
Chicken Florentine
Glazed Chicken
Grilled Chicken and Penne Pasta
Grilled Chicken Tuscan

Lifestream Waffles
Buckwheat Wildberry
Flax Plus
Hemp Plus
Mesa Sunrise

Ling Ling Potstickers
Assorted varieties

Moosewood
Broccoli and Pasta Parmesan

Nature's Path
Optimum Power Waffles

Seeds of Change
Penne Marinara
Spicy Peanut Noodles
Teriyaki Stir-Fried Rice

Shelton's
Chicken Pie
Turkey Pie

Stouffer's
Homestyle Chicken and Noodles
Spaghetti with Meatballs in Sauce

Vicolo Cornmeal Crust Pizza
Wheatstone Calzone

NUT BUTTERS

Adam's
Peanut Butter

Arrowhead Mills
Creamy Valencia Peanut Butter
Crunchy Valencia Peanut Butter

I. M. Healthy
Original Chunky Soy Nut Butter
Unsweetened Creamy Soy Nut Butter

Kettle
Hazelnut Butter

Laura Scudder's
Peanut butter

Living Tree Community Foods
Cashew Butter
Raw Sesame Tahini
Roasted Almond Butter

Maranatha
Cashew Butter
Macadamia Butter
Peanut Butter
Raw Almond Butter

Raw Tahini
Roasted Almond Butter
Roasted Tahini

Santa Fe Olé
Red Chile Peanut Butter

Trader Joe's
Calzone (chicken sausage)
Chicken Masala
Pizza Olympiad
Thai Style Green Curry

PASTA SAUCES

Amy's Premium Organic Pasta Sauce
Family Marinara
Pomodoro Zucca
Puttanesca

Barilla
Garden Vegetable
Mushroom and Garlic

Bertolli
Creamy Garlic Alfredo
Marinara with Burgundy Wine
Vidalia Onion

Classico
Alfredo
Roasted Garlic
Tomato & Basil

Newman's Own
Mushroom Marinara
Roasted Garlic & Peppers
Vodka Sauce

Prego
Garlic Supreme
Traditional

Progresso
Red Clam Sauce
White Clam Sauce

Ragú
Super Chunky Mushroom
Traditional

Seeds of Change
Roasted Garlic & Onion
Tomato & Basil
Traditional Herb

SNACK BARS

Barbara's Bakery
Nature's Choice Granola Bars
Puffins Cereal & Milk Bars

Health Valley
Apple Bakes
Café Creations
Cereal Bars
Date Bakes
Granola Bars
Tarts

Nature Valley
Chewy Granola Bars
Crunchy Granola Bars

Nature's Choice Multigrain Cereal Bars
Cherry
Raspberry

Nature's Path
EnviroKidz Organic Crispy
  Rice Bars

SOUPS

Amy's
Black Bean Vegetable
Cream of Tomato
Lentil
Minestrone
No-Chicken Noodle
Split Pea

Health Valley
Chicken Rice
Corn and Vegetable
14 Garden Vegetable
Minestrone
Mushroom Barley
Potato Leek
Split Pea

Imagine
Organic Creamy Broccoli
Organic Creamy Butternut Squash
Organic Creamy Portobella
  Mushroom
Organic Creamy Potato Leek
Organic Creamy Sweet Corn
Organic Creamy Tomato
Organic Free Range Chicken
  Broth
Organic Vegetable Broth

Pacific
Free Range Chicken Broth
Mushroom Broth
Vegetable Broth

ShariAnn's
Cream of Tomato
Great Plains Split Pea
Italian White Bean
Minestrone
Vegetarian French Onion

Shelton's
Black Bean & Chicken
Chicken Broth
Chicken Noodle
Chicken Rice
Chicken Tortilla
Chicken Vegetable

Walnut Acres (organic)
Classic Minestrone
Country Corn Chowder
Creamy Tomato
Cuban Black Bean
Ginger Carrot
Mediterranean Lentil
Savory Tomato

STOVE-TOP DINNERS

Annie Chun's noodles and sauce
Assorted varieties

Annie's Macaroni and Cheese
Shells and Real Aged Wisconsin
  Cheddar
Shells & White Cheddar
Whole Wheat Shells and
  Cheddar

Barbara's Bakery Mashed Potatoes
Deluxe Four Cheese
Kraft Macaroni & Cheese Dinner

Macaroni with Original Cheddar
    Cheese Sauce

Lundberg Organic Risotto
Assorted varieties

Patak's Tastes of India
Tangy Lemon and Cilantro Cooking
    Sauce (Tikka Masala)

Taj Ethnic Gourmet Delhi Korma
Bombay Potatoes
Kashmir Spinach

Punjab Eggplant
Simla Potatoes
Tasty Bite

Tesoros
Penne Toscana

Thai Kitchen
Thai Peanut Stir-Fry
    Rice Noodles

PERSONAL FAVORITES

Following are a few of the products I am particularly fond of, brands and products I know well and that can be found in larger markets nationwide. The cheeses listed are freshly made under the direction of the proprietors and all are wrapped for quick pickup as you shop.

Almondina
Original Biscuits
Choconut cookies
Gingerspice Biscuits
Chocolate Crunch Squares

Appel Farms
Cheddar Cheese
Feta Cheese
Quark (yogurtlike food made from nonfat, lowfat, or whole milk)

Cowgirl Creamery
Red Hawk Cheese
Organic Clabbered Cottage Cheese

Familia
Swiss Muesli (no added sugar)

Just Tomatoes
Dehydrated tomato, bell pepper, corn, peas, and carrots

Kavli
All Natural Whole Grain
Crispbread

Mazetta
Roasted Red Peppers

Thai House Prepared Sauces
Green Curry Paste
Yellow Curry Paste

Santa Fe Olé
Green Chili Sauce
Roasted Red Pepper Purée

Sensible Foods
Cracklin' Corn (contains corn and sea salt and nothing else)

Straus Family Creamery
Organic Ice Cream
Organic Plain Yogurt

Vermont Butter & Cheese Company
Chèvre
Crème Fraîche
Cultured Butter

Wax Orchards
Chocolate sauces
Chutneys

APPENDIX C

RESOURCES

Many websites, publications, and books have been particularly helpful to me in my investigation of food, fat, and history. I hope the few listed below will be equally helpful to you as you continue your exploration of the subject.

Websites

Oldways Oldways is a widely respected nonprofit food-issues think tank known for translating high-level science into consumer-friendly health promotion for consumers, health professionals, chefs, farmers, journalists, and the food industry. Oldways education programs influence government policies and reach decision makers, such as chefs and food-service executives. Oldways has developed an approach called Eatwise, which focuses on a balance of calories among carbohydrates, proteins, and fats. Contact Christopher Speed at www.oldwayspt.org for more information or to order the Eatwise consumer guide.

U.S. Food and Drug Administration Federal Register This is a great resource for staying up to date on issues under consideration by the FDA. Visit the website at www.access data.fda.gov/scripts/oc/ohrms/index.cfm.

Mary Enig, Ph.D., and Walter Willett, M.D., have contributed much to the body of knowledge about trans fatty acids and their effects on the human body. Their assistance has been invaluable in the preparation of this book.

Mary Enig, Ph.D. Dr. Enig has studied the effects of trans fats since the early 1980s. To share her knowledge of trans fats and other oils, visit her website: www.enig.com.

Walter C. Willett, M.D. Dr. Willett, chairman of the department of nutrition at the Harvard School of Public Health, and his colleagues at Harvard and around the world have extensively researched the dangers of trans fats and their effects on heart disease, primarily through the ongoing Nurses' Health Study and Health Professionals Follow-Up Study. For information on Harvard health studies, visit www.hsph.Harvard.edu

Books

Alphen, J. van, et al., and Stuyvenberg, J. H. van, ed. *Margarine: An Economic, Social, and Scientific History, 1869–1969.* Toronto: University of Toronto Press, 1969.

Critser, Greg. *Fat Land: How Americans Became the Fattest People in the World.* Boston: Houghton Mifflin, 2003.

Enig, Mary G. *Know Your Fats: The Complete Primer for Understanding the Nutrition of Fats, Oils, and Cholesterol.* Bethesda, Maryland: Bethesda Press, 2000.

Lewis, Tom. *Divided Highways.* New York: Viking, 1997.

McGee, Harold. *The Curious Cook.* San Francisco: North Point Press, 1990.

McGee, Harold. *On Food and Cooking.* New York: Scribner, 1984.

McNeal, James U. *Kids as Customers.* New York: Lexington Books, 1992.

Nestle, Marion. *Food Politics: How the Food Industry Influences Nutrition and Health.* Berkeley: University of California Press, 2002.

Rampton, Sheldon and John Stauber. *Trust Us, We're Experts!* New York: Jeremy P. Tarcher Putnam, 2001.

Ravnskov, Uffe, M.D. *The Cholesterol Myths.* Washington, D.C.: New Trends, 2000.

Schisgall, Oscar. *Eyes on Tomorrow: The Evolution of Proctor & Gamble.* Chicago: J. G. Ferguson, 1981.

Schlosser, Eric. *Fast Food Nation.* Boston and New York: Houghton Mifflin, 2001.

Simopoulos, Artemis P., M.D., and Jo Robinson. *The Omega Diet.* New York: Quill, 1999.

Tannahill, Reay. *Food in History.* New York: Three Rivers Press, 1995.

Willett, Walter C., M.D. *Eat, Drink, and Be Healthy: The Harvard Medical School Guide to Healthy Eating.* New York: Simon & Schuster, 2001.

Zeldin, Theodore. *France, 1848–1945: Politics and Anger.* London: Oxford University Press, 1979.

Publications

Eating Well magazine (www.eatingwell.com).

Environmental Nutrition, a monthly newsletter and digest of current health related issues (www.environmentalnutrition.com).

Harvard Women's Health Watch, a monthly newsletter published by the Harvard Medical School (www.health.Harvard.edu).

Inform, the journal of the American Oil Chemists Society (www.aocs.org).

Science magazine has treated the subject of fat, diet, and health in many articles. One, "The Soft Science of Dietary

Fat," by Gary Taubes (March 30, 2001), is provocative and has received international acclaim. Another, "Diet and Health: What Should We Eat?" by Walter C. Willett (April 22, 1994), offers a comprehensive look at diet and health consequences.

APPENDIX D

MEDICAL REFERENCES

Published works by medical researchers and scientists have contributed significantly to an understanding of trans fatty acids and their health effects. Highlights of some of the findings are included here. They are arranged chronologically, starting with the most recent.

Goraya,T.Y., et al. "Coronary Heart Disease Death and Sudden Cardiac Death: A 20-Year Population-Based Study," *American Journal of Epidemiology* 157(9): 763–70 (2003).

Mauger, J. F., Alice H. Lichtenstein, et al. "Effect of Different Forms of Dietary Hydrogenated Fats on LDL Particle Size," *American Journal of Clinical Nutrition* 78(3): 370–75 (2003). ". . . Consumption of dietary trans FAs is associated with a deleterious increase in small, dense LDL, which further reinforces the importance of promoting diets low in trans FAs to favorably affect the lipoprotein profile . . ."

From the Report on Dietary Reference Intakes for Energy, Carbohydrate, Fiber, Fat, Fatty Acids, Cholesterol, Protein, and Amino Acids. "Letter Report on Dietary Reference Intakes for Trans Fatty Acids," Food and Nutrition Board, Institute of Medicine (2002).

Katz, A.M., M.D. "Trans-Fatty Acids and Sudden Cardiac Death,"

Circulation 105 (6): 669–71 (2002). "The potential importance . . . is highlighted by Lemaitre et al, who in this issue of *Circulation*, suggests that dietary trans fatty acids cause sudden cardiac death . . ."

Lemaitre, R. N., et al. "Cell Membrane Trans-Fatty Acids and the Risk of Primary Cardiac Arrest," *Circulation* 105(6): 697–701 (2002). ". . . These findings suggest that dietary intake of total trans fatty acids is associated with . . . a larger increase in the risk of primary cardiac arrest. . . ."

Semma, M. "Trans Fatty Acids: Properties, Benefits and Risks," *Journal of Health Science* 48(1): 7–13 (2002).

Clandinin, M.T., and M. S. Wilke. "Do Trans Fatty Acids Increase the Incidence of Type 2 Diabetes?" *American Journal of Clinical Nutrition* 73 (6): 1000–02 (2001).

Booth, S. L., Alice H. Lichtenstein, et. al. "Effects of a Hydrogenated Form of Vitamin K on Bone Formation and Resorption," *American Journal of Clinical Nutrition* 74(6): 783–90 (2001). ". . . Hydrogenation of plant oils appears to decrease the absorption and biological effect of vitamin K in bone."

de Roos, N. M.; M. L. Bots; M. B. Katan. "Replacement of Dietary Saturated Fatty Acids by Trans Fatty Acids Lowers Serum HDL Cholesterol and Impairs Endothelial Function in Healthy Men and Women," *Arteriosclerosis, Thrombosis, and Vascular Biology* 21(7): 1233–7 (2001). ". . . Replacement of dietary saturated fatty acids by trans fatty acids impaired FMD of the brachial artery, which suggests increased risk of CHD. . . ."

Hu, F. B.; J. E. Manson; W. C. Willett. "Types of Dietary Fat and Risk of Coronary Heart Disease: A Critical Review," *Journal of the American College of Nutrition* 20(1): 5–19 (2001).

Hu, M.D., F. B.; JoAnn E. Manson, M.D.; Meir J. Stampfer, M.D.; Graham A. Colditz, M.D.; Simon Kiu, M.D.; Caren G. Solomon, M.D.; Walter C. Willett, M.D. "Diet, Lifestyle, and the Risk of Type 2 Diabetes Mellitus in Women," *The New England Journal of Medicine* 345:790–97 (2001)." . . . our findings support the hypothesis that the majority of cases of type 2 diabetes could be prevented by the adoption of a healthier lifestyle. . . ."

Kris-Etherton, P., Ph.D.; Stephen R. Daniels, M.D., Ph.D.; Robert H. Eckel, M.D.; Marguerite Enger, Ph.D., R.N.; Barbara V. Howard, Ph.D.; Ronald M. Krauss, M.D.; Alice H., Lichtenstein, D.Sc.; Frank Sacks, M.D.; Sachiko St. Jeor, Ph.D.; Meir Stampfer, M.D., Dr. P.H. "Summary of the Scientific Conference on Dietary Fatty Acids and Cardiovascular Health: Conference Summary from the Nutrition Committee of the American Heart Association/Conference Planning and Writing Committee," *Circulation* 103(7): 1034–39 (2001). ". . . Based on a large body of evidence, it is apparent that the optimal diet for reducing risk of chronic diseases is one in which . . . trans fatty acids from manufactured fats are virtually eliminated . . ."

Larqué, E., S. Zamora, A. Gil. "Dietary Trans Fatty Acids in Early Life: A Review," *Early Human Development* 65 Supplement: S31–41 (2001).

Oomen, Claudia M., et al. "Association Between Trans Fatty Acid Intake and 10-Year Risk of Coronary Heart Disease in the Zutphen Elderly Study: A Prospective Population-Based Study," *The Lancet* vol. 357(9258): 732–33 (2001). ". . . A high intake of trans fatty acids (all types of isomers) contributes to the risk of coronary heart disease. . . ."

Bhathena, S. J. "Relationship Between Fatty Acids and the Endocrine System," *Biofactors* 13 (1–4): 35–39 (2000). ". . . Saturated and trans fatty acids (TFA) decrease insulin concentration leading to insulin resistance. . . ."

Gillman, M. W., M.D., et al. "Family Dinner and Diet Quality Among Older Children and Adolescents," *Archives of Family Medicine* 9(3): 235–40 (2000)." . . . Eating family dinner was associated with healthful dietary intake patterns, including more fruits and vegetables, less fried food and soda, less saturated and trans fat, lower glycemic load, more fiber and micronutrients from food, and no material differences in red meat or snack foods."

Hornstra, G. "Essential Fatty Acids in Mothers and Their Neonates," *American Journal of Clinical Nutrition* 71 (5 Supplement): 1262S–69 (2000). ". . . Consumption of trans unsaturated fatty acids appeared to be associated with lower maternal and neonatal PUFA status. Therefore, it seems prudent to minimize the consumption of trans fatty acids during pregnancy. . . ."

Krauss, R. M., M.D., et al. "American Heart Association Dietary Guidelines: Revision 2000: A Statement for Healthcare Professionals from the Nutrition Committee of the American Heart Association," *Circulation* 102(10): 2284–99 (2000). ". . . It has been established that dietary trans fatty acids can increase LDL cholesterol and reduce HDL cholesterol . . . The AHA recommends limiting the intake of trans fatty acids, the major contributor of which is hydrogenated fat. . . ."

Lichtenstein, A. H., "Trans Fatty Acids and Cardiovascular Disease Risk," *Current Opinion in Lipidology,* 11(1): 37–42 (2000).

McGill, H. C., Jr., M.D., et al. "Association of Coronary Heart Disease Risk Factors with Microscopic Qualities of Coronary Atherosclerosis in Youth," *Circulation* 102(4): 374–79 (2000). ". . . Long-range prevention of CHD must begin in adolescence or young adulthood. . . ."

Stampfer, M. J.; M.D., Frank B. Hu, M.D.; JoAnn E. Manson, M.D.; Eric B. Rimm, Sc.D.; and Walter C. Willett, M.D. "Primary Prevention of Coronary Heart Disease in Women Through Diet and Lifestyle," *The New England Journal of Medicine* 343:16–22 (2000). ". . . Among women, adherence to lifestyle guidelines involving diet, exercise, and abstinence from smoking is associated with a very low risk of coronary heart disease. . . ."

Ascherio, A., M.D., Dr.P.H.; Martijo B. Katan, Ph.D.; Meir J. Stampfer, M.D., Dr.P.H.; Walter C. Willett, M.D., Dr.P.H. "Trans Fatty Acids and Coronary Heart Disease," *The New England Journal of Medicine* 340:1994–98 (1999). ". . . By the early 1990s it became apparent that the consumption of trans fatty acids had uniquely adverse effects on blood lipid levels in metabolic studies . . . Metabolic and epidemiologic studies indicate an adverse effect of trans fatty acids on the risk of coronary heart disease. . . ."

Ascherio, A., M. J. Stampfer, and Walter C. Willett. "Trans Fatty Acids and Coronary Heart Disease," Departments of Nutrition and Epidemiology, Harvard School of Public Health: The Channing Laboratory, Department of Medicine, Brigham and Women's Hospital (1999). ". . . Five years ago evidence was strong that trans fat had deleterious impacts on blood lipids; ensuing studies have confirmed these metabolic findings and strengthened epidemiologic support for an important adverse effect on risk of coronary heart disease. These data highlight the need for rapid implementation of labeling requirements that include fast foods. Because partially hydrogenated fats can be eliminated from the food supply by changes in processing that do not require major efforts in education and behavioral modification, these changes would be an extremely efficient and rapid method for substantially reducing rates of coronary disease. . . ."

Chandrasekharan, N. "Changing Concepts in Lipid Nutrition in Health and Disease," *Medical Journal of Malaysia* 54(3): 408–27 (1999). ". . . Trans fatty acids when compared with cis fatty acids or unhydrogenated fats have been shown to lower serum HDL cholesterol, raise serum

LDL cholesterol and when substituted for saturated fatty acids, increase lipoprotein Lp(a) level, an independent risk factor for the development of coronary heart disease. . . ."

Freedman, D. S., W. H. Dietz, S. R. Srinivasan, G. S. Berenson. "The Relation of Overweight to Cardiovascular Risk Factors Among Children and Adolescents: The Bogalusa Heart Study," *Pediatrics* 103:1175–82 (1999).

Hu, F. B., M.D.; Meir J. Stampfer, M.D.; Eric B. Rimm, Sc.D.; JoAnn E. Manson, M.D.; Alberto Ascherio, M.D.; Graham A. Colditz, M.D.; Bernard A. Rosner, Ph.D.; Donna Spiegelman, Sc.D.; Frank E. Speizer, M.D.; Frank M. Sacks, M.D.; Charles H. Hennekens, M.D.; Walter C. Willett, M.D. "A Prospective Study of Egg Consumption and Risk of Cardiovascular Disease in Men and Women," *JAMA* 281(15): 1387–94 (1999).

Koplan, J. P., et al. "The Spread of Obesity in the United States: Are Health Care Professionals Advising Obese Patients to Lose Weight?" A Report from the Centers for Disease Control, *Journal of the American Medical Association* (1999).

Kummerow, F. A., Q. Zhou, and Mohamedain M. Mahfouz. "Effect of Trans Fatty Acids on Calcium Influx into Human Arterial Endothelial Cells," *American Journal of Clinical Nutrition* 70(5): 832–38 (1999).

Lichtenstein, Alice H., D. Sc.; Lynne M. Ausman, D.Sc.; Susan M. Jalbert, M.L.T.; and Ernst J. Schaefer, M.D. "Effects of Different Forms of Dietary Hydrogenated Fats on Serum Lipoprotein Cholesterol Levels," *The New England Journal of Medicine* 340:1933–40 (1999). ". . . Our findings indicate that the consumption of products that are low in trans fatty acids and saturated fat has beneficial effects on serum lipoprotein cholesterol levels. . . ."

Lovejoy, J. C. "Dietary Fatty Acids and Insulin Resistance," *Current Atherosclerosis Report* 1(3): 215–20 (1999). ". . . Trans fatty acids appear to potentiate insulin secretion, at least in the short-term, to a greater degree than cis fatty acids. This may reflect chronic alterations in insulin sensitivity . . ."

Manson, J. E., M.D., Dr.P.H.; Frank B. Hu, M.D., Ph.D.; Janet W. Rich Edwards, Sc.D.; Graham A. Colditz, M.D., Dr. P.H.; Meir J. Stampfer, M.D., Dr.P.H.; Walter C. Willett, M.D., Dr. P.H.; Frank E. Speizer, M.D.; and Charles H. Hennekens, M.D., Dr. P.H. "A Prospective Study of Walking as Compared with Vigorous Exercise in the Prevention of Coronary Heart Disease in Women," *The New England Journal of Medicine* 341:650–58 (1999). ". . . These prospective data indicate that brisk walking and vigorous exercise are associated with substantial and similar reductions in the incidence of coronary events among women."

Morgado, N., and A. Valenzuela. "Trans Fatty Acid Isomers in Human Health and in the Food Industry," *Biological Research* 32(4): 273–87 (1999). ". . . The ingestion of trans fatty acids increases low density lipoprotein (LDL) to a degree similar to that of saturated fats, but it also reduces high density lipoproteins (HDL), therefore trans isomers are considered more atherogenic than saturated fatty acids. Trans isomers increase lipoprotein(a), a non-dietary-related risk of atherogenesis, to levels higher than the corresponding chain-length saturated fatty acid. . . ."

Srinivasan, S. R., L. Myers, and G. S. Berenson. "Temporal Association Between Obesity and Hyperinsulinemia in Children, Adolescents, and Young Adults: The Bogalusa Heart Study," *Metabolism* 48(7): 928–34 (1999).

Berenson, G., et al., "Association Between Multiple Cardiovascular Risk Factors and Atherosclerosis in Children and Young Adults," *The New England Journal of Medicine* 338:1650–656 (1998).

Hill, J. O., and J. C. Peters. "Environmental Contributions to the Obesity Epidemic," *Science* (May 29, 1998).

Rosamond, W. D., et al. "Trends in the Incidence of Myocardial

Infarction and in Mortality Due to Coronary Heart Disease, 1987 to 1994," *The New England Journal of Medicine*, 339:861–67 (1998).

Carlson, S. E., et al. "Trans Fatty Acids: Infant and Fetal Development / Report of the Expert Panel on Trans Fatty Acids and Early Development," *American Journal of Clinical Nutrition* 66(3): 715S (1997). ". . . The potential for interference with normal processes could be greatest during periods of most active cell growth, membrane expansion, metabolism, and overall developmental processes. . . . Trans fatty acids are transferred by the placenta to the fetus and incorporated into fetal tissues. . . ."

Gillman, M.W., et al. "Margarine Intake and Subsequent Coronary Heart Disease in Men," *Epidemiology* 8(2): 144–49 (1997). ". . . These data offer modest support to the hypothesis that margarine intake increases the risk of coronary heart disease . . ."

Hu, F. B., M.D.; Meir J. Stampfer, M.D.; JoAnn E. Manson, M.D.; Eric Rimm, S.c.D.; Graham A. Colditz, M.D.; Bernard A. Rosner, Ph.D.; Charles H. Hennekens, M.D.; and Walter C. Willett, M.D. "Dietary Fat Intake and the Risk of Coronary Heart Disease in Women," *The New England Journal of Medicine* 337:1491–1499 (1997). "Our findings suggest that replacing saturated and trans unsaturated fats with unhydrogenated monounsaturated and polyunsaturated fats is more effective in preventing coronary heart disease in women than reducing overall fat intake. . . ."

Willett, W. C.; Pietinen, P.; A. Ascherio; P. Korhonen; A. M. Hartman; D. Albanes; J. Virtamol. "Intake of Fatty Acids and Risk of Coronary Heart Disease in a Cohort of Finnish Men. The Alpha-Tocopherol, Beta-Carotene Cancer Prevention Study," *American Journal of Epidemiology* 145(10): 876–87 (1997). ". . . the authors observed a significant positive association between the intake of trans fatty acids and the risk of coronary death. . . ."

Gaziano, J. M., et al. "Fasting Triglycerides, High-Density Lipoprotein, and Risk of Myocardial Infarction," *Circulation* 96(8): 2520–25 (1997).

Ratnayake, W. M. N., and Z. Y. Chen. "Trans, n-3, and n-6 Fatty Acids in Canadian Human Milk," *Lipids* 31 Supplement: S279–82 (1996). ". . . our findings suggest that breast milk in Canada generally has a high level of TFA and a low level of LCP. In view of the possible inhibitory effects of TFA on essential fatty acid metabolism (6-9) and the importance of LCP for the developing brain and retina (9), the combination of high levels of TFA and low levels of LCP in milk is a cause for concern, and its possible physiological consequences on infants should be investigated."

Ratnayake, W. M. N., and Z. Y. Chen. "Trans Fatty Acids in Canadian Breast Milk and Diet," in Przybylski, R., and B. E. McDonald, eds. *Development and Processing of Vegetable Oils for Human Nutrition* (Champaign, Illinois: AOCS Press, 1996). ". . . It is well established that the fatty acids in breast milk reflect those of the maternal diet . . . the presence of TFA in human milk is a concern, because of their possible negative nutritional and physiological effects on the recipient infant. Human infants absorb and metabolize trans isomer and incorporate them into plasma and tissue lipids. . . ."

Ascherio, A., et al. "Dietary Fat and Risk of Coronary Heart Disease in Men: Cohort Follow Up Study in the United States," *British Medical Journal* 313(7049): 84-90 (1996).

Expert Panel on Trans Fatty Acids and Coronary Heart Disease. "Trans Fatty Acids and Coronary Heart Disease Risk," *American Journal of Clinical Nutrition* 62:655S–708S (1995).

Emken, E. A. "Physiochemical Properties, Intake and Metabolism," *American Journal of Clinical Nutrition* 62:659S–669S (1995).

Katan, M. B., P. L. Zock, and R. P. Mensink. "Trans Fatty Acids and Their Effects on Lipoproteins in Humans," *Annual Review of Nutrition* 15:473–93 (1995).

Chen, Z. Y.; C. Pelletier; R. Hollywood; W.M.N. Ratnayake; et al. "Trans Fatty Acid Isomers in Canadian Human Milk," *Lipids* 30(1): (1995). ". . . It is clear that trans fatty acid isomers present in partially hydrogenated vegetable oils are transferred to human milk through maternal diets and, subsequently, to infants. Feeding diets high in trans fatty acids to newborn animals led to rapid accumulation of trans fatty acids in adipose tissue, liver and heart. . . ."

Katan, M. B., P. L. Zock, and R. P. Mensink. "Effects of Fats and Fatty Acids on Blood Lipids in Humans: An Overview," *American Journal of Clinical Nutrition* 60 (6 Supplement): 1017S–22S (1994).

Judd, J. T., et al. "Dietary Trans Fatty Acids: Effects of Plasma Lipids and Lipoproteins on Healthy Men and Women," *American Journal of Clinical Nutrition* 59(4): 861–68 (1994).

Mann, G. V. "Metabolic Consequences of Dietary Trans Fatty Acids," *The Lancet* 343(8908): 1268–71 (1994).

Mensink, R. P.; E. H. M. Temme; and G. Hornstra. "Dietary Saturated and Trans Fatty Acids and Lipoprotein Metabolism," *Annals of Medicine* 26(6): 451–64 (1994).

Willett, W. C. "Diet and Health: What Should We Eat?" *Science* 264(5158): (1994).

Lichtenstein, A. H., et al. "Hydrogenation Impairs the Hypolipidemic Effect of Corn Oil in Humans: Hydrogenation, Trans Fatty Acids, and Plasma Lipids," *Arteriosclerosis Thrombosis* 13(2): 154–61 (1993).

Litin, L. and F. Sacks. "Trans-Fatty Acid Content of Common

Foods," *The New England Journal of Medicine* 329:1969–70 (1993).

Willett, W. C., M. J. Stampfer, J. E. Manson, et al., "Intake of Trans Fatty Acids and Risk of Coronary Heart Disease Among Women," *The Lancet* 341(8845): 581–85 (1993).

Pettersen, J. and J. Opstved. "Trans Fatty Acids. 4. Effects on Fatty Acid Composition of Colostrum and Milk," *Lipids* 26(9): 711–17 (1991). ". . . Feeding trans-containing fats led to secretion of trans fatty acids in the milk lipids. . . ."

Enig, M. G., S. Atal, M. Keeney, J. Sampugna. "Isometric Trans Fatty Acids in the U.S. Diet," *Journal of the American College of Nutrition* 5:471–86 (1990).

Mensink, R. P. and M. B. Katan. "Effect of Dietary Trans Fatty Acids on High-Density and Low-Density Lipoprotein Cholesterol Levels in Healthy Subjects," *The New England Journal of Medicine* 323:439–45 (1990).

Kritchevsky, D. "Trans Fatty Acid Effects in Experimental Atherosclerosis," *Federation Proceedings* 41:2813–2817 (1982).

Acknowledgments

This book began here at my desk a few years ago, one very small thought very late at night. Before the book was complete it had became a collaborative and shared effort of many physicians, scientists, and friends from universities, research institutions, and home offices around the world. Always, I was asked questions that enlarged my project and recast it freshly. There would have been no possibility of this work existing without the wisdom and generosity of this gigantic community of unseen colleagues.

To Mary Enig, I am, as are so many, indebted to you for your perseverance over so many years. Your work and determination made all our futures safer.

To Sadja Greenwood and Alan Margolis, who introduced me to the wonderland of Mesa Refuge, and to Mark Dowie, who encouraged my proposal, I am forever grateful; you know this book found its walking legs there by the Bay.

To Caroline Pincus and Suzanne Sherman, your editorial expertise and collaboration were indispensable, your judgments essential. My gratitude and appreciation seem not nearly enough.

To Micki Nuding, my editor at Pocket Books, so much appreciation for seeing this manuscript's life and, always, your wise direction during its maturing.

To David Hawkins, copyeditor extraordinaire, your

thoughtful queries and considered insights made many important differences. I am forever appreciative.

To Jeffrey Aron at the University of California Medical School, Frank Gunstone of Dundee, Scotland, Diane Meehan at Rockefeller University Hospital and her colleagues Wendy Snowdon in New Caledonia and Lois Englberger in Queensland, Australia, to Christopher Speed at Oldways Preservation Trust, and to Walter Willett and his colleagues at the Harvard School of Public Health, thank you for taking a stranger into your midst.

And always, in our ongoing beach walking and trail trudging, our phone and email conversations about love and marriage, food and writing, industry sabotage and political indiscretions, were it not for the thoughtfulness of Amanda Adelmann, Karen Archer, Charlotte Ballentine, Mary Barror, Kim Bender, Brandy Engel, Katherine Forrest, Maria Garrigues, Sadja Greenwood, Adair Heath, Paula Huntley, Lorraine Kisly, Judith Litwin, Jane Mickelson, Charles Munitz, Sheila O'Donnell, Joan Robbins, Sally Sampson, Donna Ward, Tom Williard, my daughter Sarah Shaw, my sisters Rose-Lynn Sokol and Eleanor Surkis, this book would be less than it is.

And with much love and appreciation always to my children, John, Charles, Sarah, and Lizzy, and my daughter-in-law, Lisa, who have continuously demonstrated in their kitchens that food is a matter of choice and not of habit. I hope my children will always forgive my robbing their childhood of Oreos and potato chips.

And of course, to Bob, without whose wisdom and clarity, persistence and restraint, love and humor, there would be no book.

Index

Page numbers in *italics* refer to illustrations.

Visit
❖ **Pocket Books** ❖
online at

www.SimonSays.com

Keep up on the latest new
releases from your favorite
authors, as well as author
appearances, news, chats,
special offers and more.

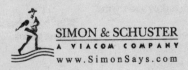